PRAISE FOR 13 WEEKS

In *13 Weeks*, Jodi Maiers captures the courage, heartbreak, and unyielding humanity that defined a generation of healers. Her words pulse with raw honesty—each page a tribute to the nurses, families, and loved ones who stood on the invisible front lines of COVID and refused to let hope die. This is not just a story of survival; it's a love letter to resilience, to the sacred calling of caregiving, and to the strength it takes to bear witness to both tragedy and grace. A powerful, soul-stirring reminder that even in our darkest hours, compassion remains the brightest light.

- Joseph J. Kochan III, M.D., Captain, Medical Corps, United States Navy

I read every chapter, every paragraph, and every word, through tears and feelings of gratitude for both Scott and Jodi for what they went through.

Reading this book, I felt like I was in the epicenter of the pandemic along with Scott. Knowing both Jodi and Scott made this book very real to me. The book hit home and stirred emotions that I had suppressed for a long time.

I felt Scott's anger, Jodi's anxiety, and the uncertainty of the COVID pandemic. I was hospitalized for three weeks in 2020 with the virus, this book brought back the raw emotions.

- Rick Cooper, RN, MSN - Retired Associate Dean of Nursing, Allegany College of Maryland

Jodi Maiers has captured the story of 2020. She wrote it in a way that reminds us all of the isolation we felt and how little we knew about anything. Her story is through the lens of her husband, a roaming nurse who actually experienced devastation firsthand. Scott wasn't assigned to Elmhurst Hospital Center in Queens. He volunteered. He could have gone anywhere, but chose to head toward the chaos of a health system that was overwhelmed, under extreme pressure, and pushed past capacity. It's the truth of a real hero and the people he left behind when he heard the call.

- Michael Allen, Author of *Joker Joker Deuce*, *The Deeper Dark*, and *A River in the Ocean*

13 Weeks is a poignant emotionally impacted true account of the worst thirteen weeks for our family during COVID. I am the mother of Scott who this story follows to New York. I can't read this without breaking into an ugly cry because it is written with such vivid and tragic recollection and of the horrors our medical heroes overcame to try and save unsavable lives.

This is a MUST read to help remind us to be forever grateful for those men and women and to also pray we are better prepared to support them for the next one.

- Joann Parker, mother of Scott Maiers

13 Weeks is a beacon, brightly illuminating the collective plight of all nurses in today's healthcare community. It is also soul-wrenchingly personal, raw, and palpably real.

I can't thank you enough for so clearly magnifying the raw demand and emotion that nurses experience every day, and for so painfully illustrating the need for mental health support as a "new norm" for these dedicated practitioners.

- Brian J. Davis, CEO of Arching Foundation, Inc.

As a fellow nurse, I was deeply moved by *13 Weeks: A Nurse's Story from the Epicenter of COVID* by Jodi Maiers. This powerful account captures the courage, compassion, and unshakable humanity of those who refused to stand by while others were suffering. When Scott said, "I can't sit here. Not while they're drowning," every nurse feels that calling—the instinct to run toward the fire, to offer comfort in chaos, to fight for life even in the darkest hours. Only a few heroes truly lived that calling, and the Elmhurst COVID warriors carry that weight; they will bear it for the rest of their lives. With honesty and grace, Maiers reminds us why we became nurses in the first place—to serve, to heal, and to stand beside our patients no matter the cost. *13 Weeks* is not just a book; it's a tribute to the resilience of the human spirit and to the extraordinary bravery of those who chose to act when it mattered most.

- Liz Henderson, RN (Momma Liz to most)

13 Weeks

A Nurse's Story from the Epicenter of COVID

Written by Jodi Maiers

13 Weeks: A Nurse's Story from the Epicenter of COVID, First edition 2025

ISBN 978-1-964445-26-7 (hardcover) 978-1-964445-24-3 (paperback) 978-1-964445-25-0 (eBook)

Book Cover and Interior Formatting and Styling by Lucie Ward

Graphics sourced on Adobe Stock

13 Weeks

A Nurse's Story from the Epicenter of COVID

Soul Spark
—PUBLISHING—

DEDICATION

To my husband, Scott and his fellow COVID Angels. You walked into the fire so others could breathe. When the world shut down, you showed up. You held the line–and in doing so, held all of us. Your courage lit the path. Your quiet strength gave me the words. This story is ours. This book is for you.

TABLE OF CONTENTS

PREFACE

Who would have thought we'd live through a moment so surreal it reads like history's darkest chapters—those we once skimmed in our history textbooks, convinced they couldn't touch our modern world? Yet here we are writing our own pages of a new history.

This book is more than words; it's heartbeat and breath, sleepless nights and fervent hopes. It's the story of my husband, Scott—travel nurse on the front lines of COVID-19—me, and of our children, our parents, our family, our peers. In these pages you'll find anger and frustration, euphoria and love, doubt and humor—and, most importantly, truth. Truth isn't always sunshine and rainbows; sometimes it's raw, ugly, gray, even painful. I've vowed to share our truth, our experience, as plainly and authentically as possible.

Just as COVID-19 was novel—"new" and previously unseen—so too was our journey. None of us had ever experienced the mental toll, the uncertainty, the isolation that would be woven through our daily lives. This story charts our pilgrimage through that uncharted territory, a world stripped of normalcy and familiarity, a family forever changed.

When I first began drafting this book, my goal was to tell Scott's story—his courage in the ICU, his longing to save lives as our world shut down, slowed down, and grew silent. But as the years passed, I realized the deeper narrative lay in what followed: the unseen wounds, the silent battles, the scars beneath our collective calm. This is that larger story—one too long overlooked by society and even by our own nursing community.

Though this is our story, countless others await their telling. My hope is that sharing ours will inspire more voices to rise, each narrative as novel and essential as the last.

INTRODUCTION

The virus had been a whisper in January, a murmur in February. But by March, it shouted.

COVID-19 was no longer a distant threat—it was everywhere. Unseen, unstoppable, reshaping the world with a force that defied borders and logic. By the end of the month, the numbers in the United States told a grim story:

- 192,301 confirmed cases
- 5,334 deaths
- All fifty states and the District of Columbia affected

Hospitals scrambled to prepare and keep up. ICU beds vanished overnight. Masks became currency. And the United States—a nation built on movement and connection—was told to stay home.

By mid-March, the virus was roaring.

New York City was the loudest. Elmhurst Hospital had become the face of the outbreak. Patients lined hallways. Nurses wept in supply closets. Refrigerated trucks idled outside, waiting for the dead. Queens accounted for 32% of New York City's cases. March 25, 2020 there were 20,011 cases citywide and 280 deaths on that day alone.

But it wasn't just New York.

Washington State had already buried its first cluster—nursing homes turned into tombs. California locked down early, trying to outrun the numbers. New Jersey and Louisiana watched their curves spike, too late to flatten. Across the country, counties began to glow red on CDC maps.

The virus didn't care about geography. It moved through airports, grocery stores, church pews, and break rooms. It found the cracks in every system—healthcare, politics, families—and widened them.

The United States was a nation unraveling in real time.

The virus didn't arrive with clarity—it arrived with confusion. Public health officials scrambled to respond, but the system fractured under pressure. States took the lead, each with their own rules, their own timelines, their own definitions of "essential." Testing was scarce. Guidelines shifted daily. The CDC said one thing, the White House another. And somewhere in the middle, frontline workers were left to improvise.

The economy buckled. Stock markets plunged in dizzying freefall. Businesses shuttered overnight. Unemployment lines stretched for blocks, crashing resource websites under the weight of desperation. Families who had never asked for help found themselves navigating food banks and stimulus forms. The word "essential" became both a lifeline and a sentence.

Social behavior turned primal. Toilet paper vanished. Hand sanitizer became gold. Masks sparked debates—first discouraged, then mandated, then politicized. Healthcare workers rationed them, stretching them for well over recommended time frames. People crossed the street to avoid each other. Elbow bumps replaced hugs. And six feet became the new measure of love.

Politically, the country split along fault lines that had long been cracking. Federal and state leaders clashed. Governors issued lockdowns while others resisted. Mask mandates were met with protests. Science became a battleground. And truth felt slippery.

This is the world that we were facing in March 2020.

CHAPTER 1

"We are now in a pandemic."

On March 13th the USA's calm façade cracked. The President's voice heard through living rooms and bars alike: "We are now in a pandemic." The single statement landed like a bomb, rewriting futures in an instant.

We're glued to the news outlets every day. New York City has been labeled as the epicenter. Cases are exploding faster than science can track and the city's hospitals are overwhelmed from the amount of patients. It is not just statistics anymore, numbers shared in the media; it is a tsunami demanding every hand on deck. It felt so unbelievable, so far away. But we knew it was coming.

Scott and I with two of our kids moved to Myrtle Beach six years ago. A dream, carefully stitched together from late-night talks and restless desire for something different, of salt-filled air, slower days, a promise of a peaceful life. For six years, it held.

Now, the dream feels like a weathered photograph curling at the edges.

My husband Scott sits at home, transfixed by the flickering TV. Each red banner of breaking news pulsates through his veins like a battle drum. ICU beds overflowing. PPE shortages. Nurses collapsing mid-shift. The screen blinks and something new is added. It blinks again. Update after update. Headline after headline. He doesn't blink back. Scott watches stoically, taking it all in.

Facebook nursing boards ignite with alarm—colleagues trading frenzied messages, case counts climbing by the minute. Sleep abandons him. He drives himself raw in the gym, punches thrown not at a bag, but at the whirl of his own anxiety. His thumb scrolls, aggressive, hungry for updates even as they tear at his mind.

"I should be there," he says, voice low, almost to himself. I don't answer. Not yet. I just watch him

Outside, the beach is quiet. A gull cries overhead. A child laughs in the distance. The world is still pretending that we aren't about to be swept away with this virus.

He turns to me, jaw clenched. "I can't sit here. Not while they're drowning."

I step forward, slowly. "You don't have to prove anything."

"I'm not trying to prove anything," he says. "I just... I know what it feels like to be in the fire. And I know what it feels like to be alone in it."

A heavy silence stretches between us, weighted with fear, expectation and resolve.

I've shared life with him for twelve years—every sunrise, every late-night laugh, every unguarded moment. I know the fierce set of his jaw, the fire in his eyes when duty calls, and I realize there's no arguing him out of this. Because it's precisely those convictions—his refusal to look away—that define him. The same selfless heart I fell in love with now drives him straight into the storm, and I can only stand by, loving him all the harder for it.

After years of chasing staffing crises across the country as a travel nurse, Scott accepted a position at Grand Strand Regional Medical Center as a PRN Super Float ICU nurse. On paper, it meant flexible scheduling—"PRN" standing for "as needed"—and floating between ICU units wherever help was short. In reality, it meant stepping into crisis, shift after shift, wherever the need was greatest. But to us, it meant something deeper. A tether. A promise. Planting roots.

We hung up the travel scrubs with quiet ceremony. Folded them, packed them away. Not because the work was done, but because we were ready to stop living out of suitcases. Ready to stop measuring time in Airbnb check-ins and unfamiliar spaces.

Scott had been traveling since 2007. I joined him in 2019. Together, we stitched our lives across state lines, hospital corridors, and midnight shifts. We learned to navigate back roads, traffic, and adapt to accents. We learned to say goodbye without flinching.

But Myrtle Beach called to us—not just with its ocean breeze, but with the idea of permanence. We longed for stability. For walls that held our pictures. For air that held the scent of our life. For something of our own.

Settling down wasn't surrender. It was peace. It was calm. It was what we were ready for.

March 22nd, eleven days after the pandemic announcement by the President, was Scott's first night at Grand Strand in Myrtle Beach SC. When he arrived for his shift, he was informed that the hospital cancelled all the PRN positions without notice or warning. He turned around and left his unit that evening with the ground beneath him firm, his steps quick and strong. This redirection was his call to action confirmed.

His fingers are confident as he swipes through his contacts, hovering over Raquel, his travel nurse recruiter. The world narrows to the space between him and Raquel. He calls. It goes straight to voicemail. A single beep—and silence. He steels himself. "Raq, it's Scott. I need to get to New York. Send me to Elmhurst [Hospital]. I'm ready to go—ASAP." His voice cracks only once, then steadies. He lets the voicemail finish, the harsh tone of recorded confirmation sealing his words. When the beep cuts off, he holds the phone away, staring at the blank screen. Now all he can do is wait—each passing second stretching into a lifetime. He knows where he needs to be. He has answered the call within.

...

The calendar catches my eye. *March 23rd. Monday.* A heavy sigh escapes—not from the usual Monday fatigue, but from something soul-deep. I feel it. I know it. I see it. I've been watching his restlessness over the past few weeks. He will not be able to stand by and watch from the sidelines. Our lives are about to change.

I arrive home after my two-hour work commute and

sit in view of our home before going inside. I need a few moments of silence and stillness to wrestle down my fear, get myself into a mental and emotional space to be understanding of whatever decision I know he's about to tell me, and harden myself for what comes next. At the door, I take a measured breath—one last grip on normalcy—then swing it open.

"Hey, Honey. How was your day?" I force the casual tone. He looks up, mouth moving soundlessly—a telltale sign I know all too well. His mind is racing faster than his lips can form the words. I smirk, half-joking as I call him out. "What's that you're saying?" He blinks, irritation flickering across his face. He straightens, trying to play it cool. I match his nonchalance. "BFF messaged me today." I tell him.

"Oh, yeah... what did she say?" He leans back, feigning casual.

The fluorescent hum of my office was a dull roar beneath my skin when my phone buzzed hours earlier. A single message from Sheila—my BFF, New York native, and fellow nurse. I tapped it open, heart thudding:

BFF: I've decided. I'm signing on as a travel nurse in New York.

A laugh almost escaped before I caught myself.

Jodi: Don't you even think about telling Scott.

Already she was firing off her reasons for making this decision and I couldn't help but respect the strength in her words. Still, I could cry knowing what she is about to walk into.

We've known each other since 2015 when we were hospice case managers. I was her preceptor. She was my new-to-hospice orientee. She called me "Windy" for my nonstop talk; she was the glorious "extra" whose laughter filled every space. We discovered our mutual obsession with bulldogs—me with my rotund, drama king, Gruxton, her with an entire canine symphony: Tank, Bocelli, Maestro, and the non-bulldogs Amati, Mozart, Fenway. We bonded over sleep-deprived twenty-four hour on-call shifts, motherhood misadventures, and a sacred girls' happy hour drinking Blue Motorcycles. Every Vroom Vroom was our battle cry, our time to laugh until we cried, vent until we were both cussing like sailors, and purge until the words were finally all used up.

Sheila's résumé sparkles: ICU neuro nurse, then hospice's guardian angel. I once painted her a future in travel nursing—kids older, adventures ahead, endless explorations.

She's eleven years younger than me and her babies are barely in grade school, so she has a bit of time before she can fall into that potential future.

And now? She plans to parachute into a pandemic. My pulse spikes at the thought. Is she absolutely insane? Dropping everything—her babies, her husband's embrace, her daily life—to walk into New York's inferno? She didn't hesitate, though. That was always her way—leaping before the ground was solid, trusting her instincts to find footing midair. I used to envy that kind of bravery. Now it terrifies me.

I imagine her in a borrowed scrubs top, hair pulled back in a messy knot, standing at the edge of a hospital hallway that smells like bleach and adrenaline. The world she's entering isn't just chaotic—it's merciless. And yet, she walks into it like it's a calling. I want to scream: *Wait. Think. Breathe.* But I know better. She's already decided. So I do the only thing I can, I become her lifeline. Her safe space. Her echo.

Jodi: You're crazy—but I've got your back. Tell me everything.

Scott already knows about Sheila's decision. I can see it on his face. He's made up his mind, even if the words haven't left his mouth yet. Telling him about hearing from Sheila today is a sideways entry into the conversation. A *I already know you're going* without actually saying it.

So I tell him. "She's decided to throw her hat in the travel nurse ring."

Scott tilts his head, playing it cool. "Oh yeah? Where?"

I see it—the flicker behind his eyes. Not a surprise. Recognition. "New York," I say, too fast. My heart thuds. "I have mad respect for her—going home now, when it's all falling apart. Pretty brave."

"I know." His voice is too even, too flat. That's when I know he's ready to tell me.

His gaze locks onto mine—steel meeting glass. No denial. No explanation. Just the quiet confirmation that everything's already in motion.

Then he speaks. Each syllable clipped, precise. Like he's rehearsed it. As if saying it cleanly will make it easier for me to hear. "I called my recruiter. Told them to send me to New York." I stop breathing. "I'm submitted to Elmhurst." The name lands like a stone in my chest. I knew it was coming. I did. I've known for weeks those words were going to come out of his mouth. I felt it in the way he moved, the way he didn't sleep, the way he scrolled like he was searching for permission. But still, I wasn't prepared.

"I talked to Shelia," he adds. "We'll split the cost of housing and go together. At least we won't be alone. We can at least have someone to talk to." I nod, but I don't know if he sees it. My throat is tight. My heart is louder than the TV on in the background.

Before I can exhale, his phone rings—shrieking through the silence. He glances down, jaw clenching, and swipes to answer on speaker.

"Hey Scott." Raq's voice cuts through the line. No warmth. No hesitation. No small talk. Urgency coming through clearly. He inhales with a resolve that both terrifies and awes me. This is it, this is the moment where there is no turning back.

"It's Raq. I got your message." A pause. "I imagine you know this already since you made the request, but Elmhurst serves one of the most diverse and densely populated areas in New York City and right now, they're reeling."

He swallows. "Okay. Then let's go." I don't know if I'm breathing. No clue how I'm still standing.

There's an extended pause, the calm before a storm. "Scott, we need to run through a few questions to complete your submission. These are automatic offers—no interview, straight deployment. Are you ready?"

He exhales. "Yes."

"You understand you'll be caring for COVID-19 patients?" "I do."

"You're accepting this assignment of your own free will?" "I am."

"You accept that you'll be exposed to COVID-19, and if infected, will have to quarantine for fourteen days—alone?" "I do."

Her voice softens just a fraction, "And if you require hospitalization, your family—your wife, your kids, your parents—won't be allowed at your side." He closes his eyes. "I do."

A final warning in her voice to get across how dire the circumstances are. "Scott, get your affairs in order before deployment. Discuss your living will, appoint a Power of Attorney or healthcare surrogate. Make sure your family knows your wishes—because once you're there, there's no turning back."

His grip tightens. "Okay. I will."

"Report to Elmhurst on April 13th," she says.

She hangs up. Deafening silence follows, I can see that he feels the weight of every word and all the miles between

Myrtle Beach and the epicenter of COVID where he's headed.

I watched him lean into the recruiter's quick-fire questions, each one sharper than the last. I froze as I listened, heart hammering, unable to believe what I'd just heard. Gone was the familiar recruiter small talk—the check-ins about spouses, the "How's the weather down there?" or "Tell me about your kids." Instead, only a stripped-down exchange, each word a surgical strike: Do you accept exposure with no cure? Are you prepared to quarantine alone for two weeks? Have you arranged your affairs in the event you fall ill?

It felt less like a career conversation and more like signing up for a one-way mission. Scott's voice—steady, practiced—did not quiver, his resolve firm. Raq, normally fashioned by years of staffing chatter, sounded raw and hurried, as if she, too, was grappling with the enormity of asking another nurse to walk willingly into a viral inferno.

I saw us all as deer caught in headlights: Scott, gripping his phone; Raq, reading off her checklist; and me, witnessing the cold calculus that this pandemic had forced upon our lives. This arrangement wasn't business as usual. It was every hope, every fear, condensed into a fifteen-minute clause. And with it came the unshakable truth: Nothing about this is normal—or anything we've ever faced before.

My voice trembled as I asked, more to myself than to him. "Do you think they're going overboard?" I needed him to laugh it off, to tell me it was all routine. He ran a hand over his smooth head, eyes dark. "I don't know," he admitted. "They have to cover all scenarios to protect themselves."

Not the reassurance I'd hoped for.

He stepped closer, earnest. "I just know I need to be there. I can't sit here watching it unfold, watching nurses pushed to their limits, patients sick and dying. I can help."

Shallow breaths stretched between us, thick with everything unspoken. Finally, I found my voice. "Then you need to go."

He circles the island peninsula in two strides and pulls me into his arms. Our hug was all at once desperate and fierce, as if it could anchor us both against the storm. I felt the warmth of a single tear tracing down my cheek.

"Please promise me you'll be safe," I whispered into his collar.

He presses his lips to my temple. "I will. We've got too much left to do for me not to."

...

Pandemic. The word echoed in my mind—hollow yet gigantic. I swallowed hard, thinking of history books and bygone eras before modern medicine. This was 2020, in America. Surely we don't need living wills for a man who lifts weights five days a week and treats his body like a temple. I couldn't wrap my head around the enormity of it. I couldn't match Scott's response. I was viewing all of this very differently than he was.

He was almost euphoric—adrenaline high, convinced he'd "save the world." His skill set was flawless: twenty-five years in ICUs, CVICU and CCU his heart's home, travel contracts all over the country. He'd been a hero in Level One traumas and tiny rural hospitals. They called him "Dr. Scott." He was the Namaste soul I married. But the storm he was rushing into? Completely novel. Unscripted. Unforgiving.

That night, we sat on the porch bathed in moonlight. I traced the tension in his jaw.

"Are you scared?" I whispered.

"No," he said, unflinching. "I've done this before. I know my protocols. I'll be fine. This is what I do."

His logic cuts through the panic like a scalpel, trying to reassure me. In the ICU, everyone will be a known risk. He'll suit up—gown, gloves, N95 masks—every motion second nature from decades of drills. He'll scrub in, scrub out, scrub in again, each step a stone in a tiny fortress against the virus he can see coming.

But I can't swallow that reassurance. Because none of this is normal. None of this is coming with a tried and true playbook. I watch him lean back, eyes steady, convinced he's covered every angle. And I feel the room tilt.

This isn't traffic duty. It isn't triage in the ER with predictable surges. This is a daily war zone with an enemy that hides in plain sight—silent, merciless. He's never faced anything like this. My chest tightens. "You haven't been here before," I whisper, disagreeing with him. But he won't really hear it, he truly believes he's prepared. He adjusts his posture. I want to shout—"It's not the same!"—but the air is thick with dread, and my voice comes out a ragged sigh.

Logic might keep him safe, protocols might shield him, but nothing can armor him against this storm's true toll. And I have no words left to stop him from walking straight into the eye of it. I grab his arm, voice trembling in the hush of our porch.

"You aren't worried at all—mentally? Do you even understand how bad this is going to be?" My words spill out, desperate. "I've seen you handle Code Blues and trauma bays, but this... this is different. Worse. I believe in your skill, but mentally, you have no idea what you're in for."

He meets my eyes, calm as ever, soothing me though I can't bring myself to hear him. My chest tightens so suddenly I can hardly breathe—each inhale shallow, each exhale a battle. My hands go clammy. I feel the world waver beneath me.

"You're allowed to be scared," I force out, panic and pleading tangled together. "Allowed to be tired, drained— allowed to feel it all in the moment. Promise me you won't try to be Superman—at least not with me."

He nods, genuine, his resolve firm. I can't shake the flutter in my gut. I swallow hard, clutch my sweater wrapping it tighter around me, and straighten my shoulders. He needs to leave without doubt, without sorrow. I press a smile to my face and whisper, "Just come back to me." And in that vow—spoken softly, fiercely against the roar of everything coming—there was a fragile truce between his courage and my fear.

Inside, my heart trembled. Can I stay strong during all of this, for all of us? Can I bury my rising panic so deeply that he never sees it? He needs zero doubt at home. He has to fight this battle unburdened by my fears.

For the first time in my life, I understand what true anxiety is. I mask it, for his sake.

CHAPTER 2

The Wind Hits All of Us

The next few days became a blur of checklists and hushed urgency. Dawn to dusk, he downloaded forms, scrolled through packing guides, and hunted down a safe apartment near Elmhurst. Every check we made felt like a countdown—each completed task edged us closer to his departure.

But the hardest tasks sat at the very top of the list—nine phone calls. Six children, his mother, my father, my sister. Nine voices waiting on the other end, each one an anchor to home.

As I sit looking at the calls we have to make I imagine saying, "He is going away to help," nine different times and the lump I'll have in my throat before each ring—how my insides will tremble as he presses "call." I'll have to steady my voice, swallow my own fears, and speak words of optimism and positivity I'm not sure I believe.I know that it is true, that he's going to help. I have full faith in his abilities. It's not the helping I'm concerned about. I know he'll be doing that. It's everything else around the helping. It's him being gone. It's him being exposed. It's him stepping into something so foreign there is no way he can prepare.

But I know our world needs people like him—mission-driven, unshakeable, determined. I can't help wondering if the world ever stops to ask what it costs though. If the world counts the tears of those left behind, trying to believe in a purpose that feels noble but hollow. We are supposed to believe that sacrifice is salvation. All I feel is the twist in my gut and the throb in my chest. It's not just fear–it's the dread that is curling around my ribs and whispering worst-case endings.

He's standing beside me, confident, steady, rubbing circles in my back as he prepares what he's going to say. We promised we'd face it together—two hearts braced against the storm, leaning on each other until the final goodbye. Because no matter how many forms we signed, no matter how neatly and organized he packed his bags, no matter how prepared he feels for what he's walking into, these calls feel like opening the gates to a new reality that we can no longer postpone.

We step out onto the porch to make the calls. It's our refuge—our safe haven. The place where conversations have ranged from hilarious to heartbreaking, from whispered dreams to unspoken fears. It's where we've sat in silence and in story, where the day begins and ends with presence.

Being outside matters. The air, the open sky, the quiet rustle of trees—this space grounds us. It calms what's chaotic. The porch has always held our truth, and it feels right to make these calls here—the ones that will be hard to get through. It steadies us when the words are heavy.

The amber glow of Edison bulbs draped across our tiny porch feel more sacred tonight. The distant fountain murmures like a lullaby. Our bulldog, Gruxton, lies full-belly spread, hind legs stretched out behind him resembling chicken wings. His sweet wrinkled face resting on his front paws—unaware his world is about to drastically change. I sit beside Scott, the weight of our secret twisting in my gut. We take one final deep breath, together, readying ourselves for the weight each word will carry.

Madison—Number Five

I call for Madison to join us on the porch. Madison is number five on our kid line of six. The only one left living at home. She comes to sit with us, barefoot and curious, her gypsy soul sensing the storm before the first thunder rolls in.

"Well, Madison," I began, voice catching, "we have something we need to tell you."

Criss-cross applesauce style, she sits on the floor, scanning my eyes and tone, reading between the words. Her energy—so fierce, so giving—throbs in the air between us. "What's going on?" she asks. "Scott's going to New York," I say, skipping the preamble. "The hospitals are overwhelmed. He's going to help."

Silence. Then, "Are you serious?"

"Yes."

Her breath catches. "That's... a lot."

I nod. "It is."

She turns to Scott, "Are you going to be safe?" Then back to me, "Are you okay?"

She doesn't ask about logistics. She asks about *us*. That's Madi.

Scott jumps in seeing her worry increasing. "I'll be careful. I've got the gear. I'll be trained. I'll be okay."

Her gaze widens with the gravity of it all. No additional words are needed—she has absorbed every dire headline, every urgent plea on the endless news loops, and our constant COVID conversations. The downfall of being a child of nurses. Tears slide down her cheeks. She stands, crossing the distance in two strides, and wraps Scott in the tightest hug I'd ever seen.

"I know you will," she says, but her voice shakes. "I just hate that this is happening. I hate that you have to go. I'm so proud of you. I love you so much."

Her selflessness glowed like the porch lights around us—steady, warm, unmistakable. Madison, our lifelong cheerleader—pom-poms in hand since she was little—had always known how to rally a team. But her truest cheers were never shouted from sidelines. They were felt in the quiet ways she showed up for us, again and again. Tonight, she was giving her heart to someone else's crisis, just as she'd always done for ours. What she didn't know yet was that this moment marked the beginning of something deeper.

The porch swayed with its familiar calm—but tonight, the peace felt fragile. After she left, Scott and I sat in the hush she left behind. No words passed between us. We didn't need them. What lingered in his eyes mirrored what stirred in mine: pride, ache, and the quiet knowing that something had shifted. Madison had stepped into something bigger than she realized. She didn't yet know the magnitude of what was unfolding—not just the daily fear we'd carry for Scott, but the emotional terrain she'd help me navigate. She was about to become my rock. My safe place. The one who will hold space for my unraveling while helping me stay whole.

Garrett—Number Two

Scott opens his phone and pauses on a single photo—his thumb hovering over a face filled with a carefree grin. In the image, Garrett is leaning against a cruise ship railing, tie-dyed shirt bright as a summer sky, mirrored sunglasses perched on his nose, long dark hair tumbling around his shoulders. That translucent moment of joy—no pandemic worry—feels like a lifetime ago.

He lets out a soft breath, tapping the picture to call. I hear the ring and take a steadying breath. This was Garrett—our wise, ever-present number two on the kid list, the one whose laughter during 3 a.m. debates still echo through my thoughts.

"Hey, Bud. What are you up to?" Scott's voice was careful, almost light.

"Hey, Dad," came Garrett's half-awake reply. "What's going on?"

Scott exhaled. "I need to talk to you about something."

Now with hesitance he replies, "Okay..."

"This virus is getting worse." Scott says.

Yeah..." Garrett's voice barely held. It drifted out like a sigh he couldn't catch, thin and frayed at the edges.

"Well, it's hit New York hard. I've decided I need to go help."

I've often wondered how it is that silence can be so loud. When the moments between words are roaring with everything felt and unsaid.

Garrett is now very present in this moment.

A massive sigh comes through the line. "Okay."

I feel a cold anger rise at Scott's gloss-over—his refusal to name what this really means for Garrett. Doesn't he see it? Garrett needs the full truth, not softened edges. I cut in, slicing through the haze with clarity. No room for vagueness. Not now. "Garrett, your dad and I have talked through the worst. If something happens—quarantine, hospitalization—you might need to step in. Do you understand this?"

I didn't want to sound so harsh, but we need to be clear. Still, my heart aches. I press my palm to my heart, it's pounding like a warning drum. My chest is heaving. My words to Garrett sting my own ears and I hate myself for the burden I just dumped on him. I close my eyes and will myself to breathe. In...out... When I open my eyes, I adjust myself in my chair and tuck in my fear. It's time to don the "momma mask." Teeth together, spine straight, dry eyes, breaths even. I lean into a facade of calm.

I continue, "I'm proud of him—for stepping up, for helping patients and his fellow nurses when they need him most. We need him, but right now, so many others need him more. It wouldn't be fair to deny them his gift." It's true but it tastes like a lie because I don't want to accept it. It tastes bitter, like raw kale or arugula, but it shields my breaking heart.

I hold my breath.

Garrett's voice breaks through, warm and assured: "Dad, I'm proud of you, and I'm going to miss you. Promise to keep in touch."

Scott chuckles—because getting a timely text from Garrett requires more coaxing than starting an IV on a restless patient. "Thanks, Buddy. You know you'll always be my main man. I love you. We'll come out for dinner for Jodi's birthday. See you then."

The certainty in Scott's words are like a lifeline—quiet, firm, and unadorned. No tears. No trembling. The kind of strength that holds you together.

I feel a flicker of relief. But also something sharper: a brief, unwanted stab of disappointment on Scott's face. He'd braced for grief, for an avalanche of emotion—and instead found stoic tenacity.

Scott may have hoped for more emotion from Garrett, but he is exactly who we need him to be right now: resolved, understanding, steady. Still, I know him. And I worry that beneath the calm, he's absorbing more than he shows—carrying the weight quietly, not just for his dad, but for all of us.

As Scott sets his phone on the table and rubs his head, I wonder how deep a toll this is taking on him. I wonder if he ever thought he'd have to have this conversation at this stage of his life. This was an end-of-life conversation, a what-to-do-if-I'm-unable conversation, not generally one you have in your late forties when you're in great health.

Two down, seven more to go. And next, we call Scott's mother.

Momma Jo—Scott's Mom, AKA, Nan to our kids

His mom answers the phone, her voice is familiar and warm, then quickly turns tight and filled with tension after Scott breaks the news.

"What did you just tell me about this virus?" she demands. Her words come fast, urgent.

Scott's tone sharpens in response. "Mom, I'm doing what I need to do. You taught me this. You and Eddie helped anyone and everyone—whenever you could, even when you couldn't. I can't sit here while nurses are hurting, tired, over-worked. I have to go help. It's gotten worse in New York and I *am going to help.*"

Before he finishes, her scream cuts through the night—raw, blood-curdling. Then come the sobs, crashing over the line like waves.

Scott exhales, irritation flashing in his voice. But I reach for his hand, grounding him.

"Momma," I say, voice steady, "we know how much you worry. He's trained for this. We've arranged every precau-tion—PPE, quarantine protocols, daily check-ins."

Her sobs soften into quiet listening. We promise her that we'll call every day, share every update.

When the line finally clicks off, her final, *"I can't do this,"* echoes in my ear. I close my eyes, fighting back my own tears . As a mother I understand her pain.

Scott reaches out, placing his hand on my leg, gently squeezing—reminding me of his strength. I meet his gaze, and the world narrows to just the two of us—sitting on this porch under the flickering amber glow of the lights,

Gruxton's warm body pressed against my leg.

"I'm sorry," I whisper, voice thick. "She's just scared."

He presses my hand. "I know."

But I know he wanted something else. He wanted her to say what the kids have said: *"I'm proud of you."*

Except that word feels like a cruel oversimplification and not something his mother is capable of expressing right now. She's in shock. She's heartbroken. She's worried. Her worst fears as a mother are now a very real potential. Her son is putting himself directly in the middle of this untamable outbreak and we have no assurances that he'll survive. So, proud. Yes, she's proud. We all are. We know the courage and bravery that it takes for Scott to do this. But to set aside everything else and focus on our pride in him, that's just too much to ask right now.

"We need to call Kailee next," I said to keep us moving through the calls. His mom's call was hard and they won't get any easier.   We take another moment and then we steel ourselves for the next call.

Kailee—Number Three

Kailee—twenty-four, number three on the kid list. I call her Fancy, a nickname she loathes but earned. Everything about her is Fancy—her personality, her attitude, her appearance.

She mirrors me more than either of us care to admit.

She'd been here with us a week ago, visiting for her annual Spring Break trip—the one we count down to like it's Christmas. Usually, it's Starbucks runs, acai bowls, beach days, and market hauls for all the Fancy essentials. But this year, her visit was different. This year, Nan, along with the pandemic, arrived with her.

During her week here, the news grew scarier. Glued to her Facebook feed, absorbing every headline, every comment thread, every shared article, Nan's updates grew more urgent. South Carolina hadn't issued a stay-at-home order yet, but the warnings were everywhere.

Still, Scott and I clung to routine—gym sessions, masked and distanced. For him, it was therapy. For me, a break from chaos. But Kailee saw through it.

She argued. "It's not a good idea. Going to the gym for vain reasons isn't worth it. They're telling us to stay home unless we have to go out. The gym isn't a *have to.*" All said in true Fancy fashion. This time, she was absolutely right.

We tried to reassure her. She wasn't having it. "You're being stupid and selfish," she snapped. "You're telling us to take this seriously, wiping down the damn walls, but you think it's okay to go to the gym?" She stormed off to the bedroom.

And though we didn't admit it then, we knew she was right. We were clinging to a false sense of security. Somewhere deep down, we believed: *We're in the USA. We're special. We're immune. Everyone is overreacting. A few days, maybe. A couple weeks at most. It will be all good.* Now we had to call her. Now we had to admit she was justified in her fears. We are not special. We are not immune. This is real and now everything is different.

...

As of March 27, 2020, COVID-19 in the US is progressing rapidly. Approximately 86,000 confirmed cases with approximately 1,300 deaths. This period marked the beginning of widespread awareness and public health responses, including social distancing measures and stay-at-home orders in many states. New York State reporting approximately 37,000 confirmed cases. Roughly 25,000 confirmed cases in New York City alone, the majority within the state. Deaths in New York state: around 300 with New York City accounting for a significant portion of these fatalities. It's at this time that New York has become the epicenter of the pandemic in the United States.

...

We're sitting here on the porch in these captain chairs that we bought in Florida. I inwardly attempt a chuckle as I realize they are the perfect metaphor for this evening. Scott's chair is sturdy, in great shape, with a solid and supportive side table. My chair is a bit more delicate, fragile, and petite with the side table dangling haphazardly off the side. Scott is holding together, I'm barely holding on. Meanwhile, Gruxton snores at our feet, thankfully blissfully unaware.

Scott dials. Kailee picks up after a few rings. "Hey Fancy, what are you doing?" I ask, trying to sound normal.

"Not much," she replies, frustrated. "Just working and studying, waiting to see when we're supposed to go back to school."

We exchange small talk—work, school, the usual. Then I shift. "So... we have something we felt you needed to hear from both of us."

"Okay," she says, curious.

"Scott has decided to go to New York to help with the pandemic." I hold my breath.

"Wow, really? Scott, are you sure? I mean, I'm proud of you and respect you for wanting to go, but are you sure?

Are you scared? Where in New York?" Her questions tumble out, one after another, no time to answer.

"Mom, how do you feel? Are you going with him? What's Madi going to do?"

"I'm submitted to Elmhurst," Scott begins. "In Queens. Staffing is overwhelmed. I feel like I need to go help. I can't just sit here knowing that. Your mom's not going," he adds. "She's safest here."

I flinch. Like I don't have a choice. He's decided and that's final. I am a little irritated, but also feel grateful. It's true. I am safest here and he doesn't expect me to run into this. Regardless, he's not worried about his own safety. That is apparently something I need to carry. My emotions are all over the place. Every word feels like it has a deeper meaning. Yes, I am safest here, but so is he. My rollercoaster of emotions is exhausting.

"My skillset isn't needed right now," I add. "I won't go into a setting where I'd be a hindrance. If and when that time comes, I'll reassess."

Kailee pauses. Then her voice softens. "Wow. I'm proud of you. I love you. And honestly, I wouldn't expect anything less of you. Be safe." An audible breath then, "Mom," she says with so much compassion, "if you need anything, you let me know. I love you too."

Taylor—Number Four

The one reaction that completely caught us off guard

Taylor—number four on the kid line. Her whole life, she's been the quiet one. The one who flows with the current, no matter how rough. Smart, funny, private. She never complains. She never asks for much.

Scott taps the "Taylor" icon on his phone. "Hi Honey, what are you doing?" he asks.

"Nothin'." Her usual reply. We've learned she opens up more when we gently pry.

After the typical small talk—school, her day, a few laughs—I give Scott the look. Now's the time. He shifts in his chair, posture upright, leg bouncing like a sprinter at the starting line. "The virus is getting bad," he begins. "Hospitals are needing staff..." He pauses. "I've decided to go to New York and help..." Another pause. "And I wanted you to hear it from me, and see how you felt about it."

Silence.

Then sobs.

Her sobs.

We look at each other—stunned. This, we hadn't prepared for. Not from Taylor.

It's not that we thought she didn't care. She's just private. Masterful at containing emotion. But this—this was uncontrolled.

"Honey, it's okay. I'm going to be okay," Scott says, trying to comfort her.

For the first time since all this began, I don't bristle at his reassurance. Taylor needs her dad to be strong. I don't know if she's been watching the news or tracking the numbers. Her reaction doesn't need context. It's pure. It's real.

"It's only thirteen weeks," he continues, giving her more and more information hoping that it helps settle her emotions. "Then I'll be home. Jodi's staying here, working in Charleston. She'll be safe—she won't be out seeing patients. I'm leaving April 12th and starting on the 13th, so... there's not enough time to come visit before I go."

I press my palms flat against the arms of my chair. The condensation from the humid night grounds me. This latest truth crashes in painfully: He won't see all the kids before he leaves. I hadn't even considered that.

We've always carved out time to visit all of them before leaving on assignments. Now, airport rules and infection fears, plus the short timeline, have stolen these moments from us. Tears threaten once again, but I hold them back.

This isn't the time. He needs me to keep it together. Our kids need me to remain strong through this.

All the information and specifics from Scott didn't help. Taylor was not comforted. I feel like her reaction most closely mirrors my inner turmoil. All three of us are exhausted by the time we end the call.

As the night goes on, and we make one call after another, I start channeling the universe—pleading for protection, peace, clarity. I know I won't be able to get through this on my own. I see a lot of prayers in my future. For all of us.

Zach—Number Six

Zach, the baby of the family. Number six of six. A junior in high school, navigating this chaos with his own disruptions. His baseball season—postponed. School—now virtual. His world, once predictable, now uncertain. Knowing this, we tread lightly. His plate is already full.

"Hey buddy," I say, summoning my most normal voice.

"Hey Mom," he replies. "What are you doing?"

"Not much. I hear school went virtual, and baseball's postponed. How are you feeling about that?"

"I don't know," he says, voice uncertain. "I just hope we can have baseball. But it's out of my control, so I'm just trying to do the best I can."

I hear his disappointment even through his best efforts to disguise it. Baseball is his dream—his path forward. He knows what losing a season could mean. But I also hear his effort to stay grounded. To control what he can. To let go of what he can't. He's growing up faster than he should have to. And it breaks my heart.

"Scott and I wanted to talk to you about something."

"Okay..." he pauses. "What?"

"As you know, the virus is getting bad. Hospitals are begging for help. New York is being hit hard, and Scott has decided to go there and help." Again, the words spill out without breath.

"Wow, okay," he replies, hesitant. I can't tell if he doesn't believe it, or just doesn't know what it means. I debate how much to say. Scott reads me and takes the lead.

"Well Bud, we're not sure of much right now. It's serious, but I'm going well prepared and will be safe. I'll be home in thirteen weeks. In the meantime, you can text or call me whenever—I'd like that."

"Are you scared?" Zach asks, soberly.

"No, I'm not. I know what I need to do, and I'll take every precaution."

"I love you, Scott."

"I love you too, Buddy."

There is definitely something wonderful about still being young. You're better able to roll with the punches, take things at face value, and absorb what you're being told without it getting too emotional. Zach, while obviously concerned and aware of the danger, took it in stride. Perhaps there is a lesson that I can learn from him.

Jordan—Number One

Jordan, the oldest. Number one on the kid line. We brace ourselves for another call. Sometimes, I wish they wouldn't answer.

"Hey Honey," I say, voice carefully composed.

"Hey Mom," he replies, casual.

"How are you doing with all the new restrictions? Are you still able to work?"

"No, they had to close. Just waiting to see for how long." Frustration lingers in his tone.

"Well, I'm not unhappy about it," I say. "I think it's the safest thing right now for all of us. Which brings me to the reason for calling." I glance at Scott.

"Hey Jordan," he begins. "Just wanted you to hear it from me. I'm going to New York to help out with the virus. They're hurting for staff. Numbers are bad up there." He finishes with that now-familiar nonchalant save-the-world tone. It's really starting to wear on me. Why can't he stop—just for a minute—and see this isn't just another assignment.

"Oh wow, really," Jordan replies. Jordan's always been a person of few words, even as a child. Even keeled. Unmoved by hype. His reaction is expected—but still disappointing. He, like Scott, doesn't seem to grasp the severity. The implications. The cost. I'm starting to wonder if I am overreacting. My gut—still lodged in my feet even after all these days—says no, I am not overreacting.

"Yeah," Scott continues. "I contacted my recruiter and told them to send me to New York. The need is desperate. I'm trained. This is what I do."

"Wow, that's crazy," Jordan says. "Be safe. Let me know how it goes."

"I will."

"I love you."

"I love you guys too," Jordan ends.

My Dad and Jackie, my sister

Calling my dad and my sister, Jackie, brings a slight glimmer of relief—but uncertainty clings to it. Relief, because they've always been my support system. Uncertainty, because I'm not even sure what I expect of them—how they'll carry this with me, how long they'll be able to. And maybe that's the hardest part—needing them more than ever, while fearing I'm asking too much.

Scott heads inside while I make this call to give me some space. He knows my emotions are going to come pouring out as soon as Jackie answers. I can't hide any part of myself from her. Uneasiness settles within me as I get ready to call her. I'm adding to her burdens, and she already carries more than most. It feels unfair. But I need her now more than ever.

She picks up on the second ring. "Hey Sista," she says, voice amiable but tired. I swallow the lump in my throat.

"Hi Sister. I need to tell you something." There's a pause. She knows me well enough to hear the emotion I'm trying to hide.

"What's going on?"

"Scott's going to New York," I say quickly, like ripping off a waxing eyebrow. "To help with the virus." Silence. Then a sharp inhale. "Oh, Jodi..."

"I didn't want to drop this on you," I say, already apologizing. "You have enough on your plate. But I needed you to know. I need you."

"When?" she asks as though she's bracing for impact.

"He leaves April 12th." I say with an exhausted sigh. I

still can't believe it.

"Damn." She exhales slowly. Then, softer, "Are you okay?"

I want to say yes. I want to be the strong one. But I can't lie to her. "I don't know," I admit. "I'm trying to be. For the kids. For him. For his mom. For Dad. But I feel like I'm holding my breath, and I don't know when I'll get to exhale."

Jackie is quiet for a moment. Then she says, "You're not alone in this. You hear me? You're not." I nod, even though she can't see me. Her words wrap around me like a weighted blanket—heavy, grounding, necessary.

"I just keep thinking," I whisper, "what if something happens and I'm not there?"

"You *are* there," she says firmly. "You're holding the line at home. You're keeping the kids steady. You're giving him the strength to go. That's not nothing." I blink back tears. She always knows how to find the truth buried beneath my fear.

"I'm scared," I say.

"I am too," she replies. "But we'll get through this. Together. Tell Scott I love him and am so proud of him and to be safe. I've got you, Sista. Whatever you need."

We hang up, and I sit in the quiet for a long time. Jackie

didn't flinch. She didn't crumble. She absorbed the weight and stood taller, just like a big sister is expected. And somehow, that gives me permission to breathe—just a little.

It's late and we are tired but we have one last call to make.

"Hi Dad," I say, skipping the small talk. "Scott is here with me and we wanted to call and let you know—he's has decided to go to New York to help with the virus."

"Okay," he replies, matter-of-fact. "When?"

"I'll leave on April 12th," Scott tells him.

"Is it safe?" Dad asks, shifting into his well-used "dad voice" that I am grateful for right now. The tone and cadence is familiar, reassuring. There is safety in hearing it.

Scott answers calmly. "It's what I do. I've worked in isolation before. I know the precautions. They say there's plenty of PPE now, but I'm bringing my own just in case."

Dad shifts the conversation to me. "So, Jodi..." He only uses my name when it's serious. Usually it's Buckwheat or My Darling Daughter.

"What are you going to do? Are you going too?" His tone shifts—now laced with worry. "No, Dad," I begin, fabricating strength. "I'm staying at my job in Charleston. We talked it through and considering all the unknowns it's safer for one of us to be home for the kids. God forbid he gets sick—I won't be able to be with him. None of us will. But we decided this is where I need to be. At least one of us should be here."

"I can't have her getting sick," Scott interjects. "It's safer for her to stay. She has minimal contact with people. No patient exposure."

My knight in shining armor. I feel my heart flutter when he says it. But I can't deny the flicker of guilt that I'll be staying safe while he's running off to be in the middle of it all.

"I agree with that," Dad replies, relieved. "You be safe. I'm proud of you. Thank you for your service. I love you, and I'll be praying for your safety and health," he tells Scott.

I'm a mix of contradictions right now. Frustrated that he's going on his own, that I'm not "allowed" to go. But also relieved that I can't go, that I will be here where it's safer. But the reality is that my kids will still have their mom safe and protected and his kids are losing their dad to the unknown and uncertainty of what he'll be facing. My dad thanks his lucky stars I'm not the one walking into the fire. His Mom weeps in fear. No matter how may times Scott says he has PPE, that he's trained for this-none of us are reassured. Because training doesn't promise survival. And gear doesn't guarantee goodbye won't come too soon.

Nine calls done. Nine emotional landscapes traversed. Each call brought a different voice, a different reaction. Some are stunned. Some are angry. Some are quiet, trying to find the right words and failing.

Scott's decision to go to Elmhurst is rippling outward, touching people who love him, people who depend on him, people who never imagined he'd walk straight into the fire. Everyone experiences this differently. Some want to talk him out of it. Some want to thank him. Some just want to understand.

And while Scott prepares to leave, I'm left managing the aftermath from home—fielding questions, soothing fears, trying to hold space for everyone else while barely holding myself together.

Beneath it all, this truth remains: it's not about ego or accolades. It's not even about saving the world. Scott is answering a call he's carried in his bones since the moment he held his first patient's hand. His nursing heart has grown restless—pacing at the edges of routine, aching for purpose. This is where he finds meaning. This is the man I love. So even though I have no idea how I'll navigate the weeks ahead—how I'll wake each day with purpose, how I'll be the strength our family needs—I will. Because this is who he is. And loving him means honoring the call, even when it terrifies me.

My role now is to be his anchor. To be the calm in the center of this storm. He's not the only one affected by his decision. We all are. We're all a part of what he's walking into. The raging wind will hit us all. None of us are coming out of these next thirteen weeks the same as we are today.

CHAPTER 3

No Longer About Me

APRIL 2020. TEN DAYS UNTIL HE LEAVES.

April 1, 2020, COVID-19 in the U.S. is rapidly worsening. New York State reporting confirmed cases surging to approximately 130,000. New York City alone has approximately 60,000 confirmed cases. The death toll in New York State is rising over 4,500, with New York City accounting for a large proportion of these fatalities.

Nationwide, the U.S. is reporting over 200,000 confirmed cases.

I barely remember closing my eyes now the alarm shrieks bringing me back to reality. Sleep is eluding me these days. My waking hours are consumed with COVID. My mind bounces between thoughts and questions without any resolution. How it will impact us all personally. What Scott is walking into. How the world is dealing with it. All the people who are getting sick and the horrifying amount who are dying. Still, the first thing I do every morning is turn on the news. It drones on hour after hour, a never ending backdrop to my days. I lay there a beat too long, listening to the latest news. Infection rates. What the officials are saying. How the hospitals and staff are coping. Finally, I peel myself out of the bed, stumble into the kitchen, and brew coffee strong enough to cut through fog.

Porch light on. Laptop open. Phone and coffee in hand, my morning ritual unfolds: Check work emails—urgent alerts, policy updates, another round of mandatory Zoom trainings. Scroll social feeds—endless feeds of fear, "essential worker" badges, friends posting memes to ease the tension. I sip my coffee, trying to taste something other than dread as I prepare for my day ahead.

The two hour drive into work is apocalyptic with empty roads and shuttered shops. It's just me and the radio. My heart drops with each news bulletin. I scream at the car speakers. "This can't be real!" Even though it's been weeks, it still feels so surreal. Each day is getting worse making it even more difficult for the reality of it all to sink in. And everyone is still speculating. No one knows how to handle any of this. My "best guesses" about COVID feel more reliable than any official report.

It's April 1st. I glance at the calendar and sigh. April. "Me Month," I mutter under my breath. "Happy Fucking Me Month." I decided this year to tone down my birthday month, it's the best defense against disappointment. With Scott leaving in just over a week I don't feel like celebrating anyway.

Part of me envies the mission-driven, adrenaline-fueled days that Scott has in his job. He moves through his days with purpose, each hour a battle, each shift a reckoning. There's clarity in crisis. Urgency. Meaning. He gets to see the results of the work he does. So while he is prepping to head to Elmhurst and getting ready for the storm he's heading toward, I am leashed to my desk. Half-listening to slides about compliance and cleaning protocols, clicking through reminders to sanitize keyboards and avoid communal coffee pots. Each slide feels like a slow bleed—death by PowerPoint.

When the final Zoom meeting finishes, I lean back, grateful this work day is over. I close my laptop and breathe a prayer: "Keep us safe. Give me the strength to mask my fear until he's back home again." He hasn't even left yet and I'm already praying for strength to get through these next thirteen weeks. I have been furiously speaking into the universe, begging for his safe return and the shielding of his soul.

My days right now are bracketed by time on the porch. It is my only place of solace right now. The muted glow of the Edison lights, the soft sound of morning and evening insects chirping their tunes, and the fresh air give me a bit of comfort in a world that suddenly feels like it's spinning out of control. My days are full of chasing some kind of clarity through headlines, forging calm in tiny rituals, and praying my way toward strength. But tonight, once I get home, I'll let the quiet remind me that we're still here, still breathing, still holding onto hope that things will be as Scott predicts. Manageable. Prepared. Helpful.

After my hours-long drive home there is something to break up the worry and routine to look forward to. Madison is home and hinted at something planned for me.

"Happy Me Month, Momma!" she calls out, her sunshine-and-confetti energy bursting through the door before I can even set down my bag. Her grin is contagious, tugging me out of my funk as she circles me. Her joyousness reminds me how this all began—birthdays reborn as Me days, sacred pauses to celebrate ourselves.

When I turned forty, I claimed the whole month. Me Month became my unapologetic ritual: daily indulgences, social media countdowns, donut runs, full-face makeup, and Scott's legendary cheesecake. My family played along, eye rolls and all, knowing it was my way of reclaiming joy.

But this year, the joy feels borrowed. I used to beg the Me-Day gods for sunshine, tracking weather apps like a pilgrim chasing prophecy. Rain felt like betrayal. And tonight, the sky is clear. I lift my face and feel a quiet warmth—not from the sun, but from within. The kind that comes from knowing who I am, where I've been, and who still stands beside me. Scott is still here. For now. And that alone is worth celebrating.

"Ahh thanks Honey," I say with forced excitement.

"I can't wait to give you your present," she exclaims with Scott sheepishly grinning in the background. They are clearly up to something which in previous years would fill me with delight. But this year, I just can't muster the excitement I know they're expecting from me.

"I can't wait either," I half-heartedly reply. I come face to face with my sweet child and husband grinning ear to ear.

Laying on the counter is a yellow index card that reads, "Today is your Me Day and because we are quarantined, I came up with this scavenger hunt for the birthday QUEEN!" After following ten canary yellow, handwritten, poetic index card instructions I come to the finale. On her bed I see balloons, gifts, and her computer opened. I am overwhelmed and trying very hard to contain my emotions. On her computer is a video of birthday wishes that she secretly asked friends and family to send. I have never been so moved by such thoughtfulness in my life. She and my husband, with everything else that is going on, managed to make my Me Day all about me.

...

Our ritual road-trip before each new contract will look different this time. Travel bans have locked down I-95, and the urgency of his departure leaves no room for mapping out detours or goodbyes. We'll have to settle for FaceTime and phone calls with family who are scattered too far away to reach. Thankfully we have Madi, who lives with us and Garrett, just a few miles away.

APRIL 11, 2020.

Tonight was dinner at Garrett's. The meal wound down beneath a violet sky, the air thick with the unspoken awareness that these were our last few moments together before Scott leaves. We lingered over steak plates, sighing as if each breath might slow time. Garrett's laughter tangled with Frog's panicked strut, his personality-driven rooster darting through the yard in playful sprints—a memory we all wanted seared into our hearts. It felt like trying to memorize a sunset. Knowing it would fade, but watching anyway. Concentrating to remember every hue.

When the dishes were stacked and the guacamole gone, we lingered in the kitchen, wiping already-clean counters— anything to delay goodbye, to stay close a little longer. I hug Kelsey, Garrett's girlfriend, who has been part of our family for over three years. Garrett and Scott continue now with their eleventh or twelfth wipe of the counter. Madi is standing watching this unusual scene, unsure of what to do. Her discomfort at this parting is more easily detected; she isn't good at hiding. I cling to Garrett telling him I love him. Madi approaches, hugs Kelsey and they giggle about something trivial and tell each other to be safe. She turns to Garrett, him being the protective brother, informs her that she *will* be safe at work, while they hug their goodbyes. She sinks into him and he engulfs her—his arms have always been her safety net. Scott and Garrett meet in the center of the kitchen. Meanwhile, us girls start wiping the now sparkling clean counters again, watching father and son say their goodbyes.

They speak quietly to each other. Scott's voice drops into the softest dad-voice I've ever heard from him. "I love you, Bud. You'll always be my main man." Garrett's words are muffled and his body quivers in Scott's embrace. Garrett, who is taller than Scott, is a grown man with a strong, muscular stature, but with this tremulous goodbye I see a scared little boy. He's shaken, fearful, and uncertain. They embrace harder, longer. I feel the pounding of my heart in my ears. Their cries are soft, originating in their souls. Assurances that Scott will be safe. Promises that he'll see Garrett in July. And that's it. We leave, and I know that Scott and Garrett are taking a piece of each other with them.

The drive home from Garrett's takes forty minutes. We don't speak—just sit with our thoughts, heavy and unspoken. I wish I could keep driving, the way we kept wiping clean counters. It's not about the task—it's about postponing what's next.

While driving home, my mind replays all the memories

we've made since moving to Myrtle Beach. The Mellow Mushroom, where Garrett had his first Myrtle Beach job, the best pizza in town. Captain George's, Madi's first job and the best seafood buffet on the beach. Carolina Ale House where we had Madi's graduation dinner there. Four years of cheering on our MadiB and the Sea Sea Haawwwks! We drive by Market Commons fields where Zach played baseball and learned the hard way what "Big Boy Chap" was. His poor thigh area chafed so badly playing in polyester baseball pants for thirteen hours during the hot South Carolina summers. All the beach days on 48th Avenue that made it feel like endless summers. Garrett and Fancy's 21st birthday celebrations happened here in Myrtle Beach. Garrett's band debut was here. We've lived a life here, we all have. It brings a bittersweet smile to my face

We continue driving and I see the beautiful Myrtle Beach skyline with the SkyWheel and towering hotels. It never gets old. When we moved here six years ago, we were told that it would and eventually we'd stop noticing it, that our exuberance for this place would wear off. It hasn't, it's only gotten better. And now I am clinging to this place where we've built a life to sustain me while Scott is away.

CHAPTER 4

Departure Day

The countdown has expired. Today is the day. April 12, 2020. He is all packed. The truck is loaded and gassed up for the nearly twelve hour drive to his temporary apartment in New York that he'll share with Sheila, BFF. He decided to get an early start so he has time to unpack and unwind and mentally prepare before orientation tomorrow.

Coffee this morning is quiet and solemn. Again, I ask for what feels like the hundredth time, "Are you scared?" And again, his response is stoic and protective, "I'm not, I know what to do, I've been in isolation rooms before. I will take all precautions. I need you and the kids to do the same. Keep with your workouts, you can do them at home and promise to continue to eat healthy." I concede to his request with intention to follow through as this is something that is very important to him. I mean, it's the one thing I can do while he is battling COVID on the front lines.

He rises from his chair on the porch, kisses me on the forehead, and heads inside the house to pack the last necessities. The air is heavy which mimics my heart. And by the way his movements appear, he is heavy too, although unwilling or unable to admit it. His heaviness and mine are completely different. He's focused on the long drive and settling in somewhere new, being away from all of us, learning a new staff and hospital, and then facing all the COVID unknowns. My heaviness is pretending that I'm not scared, that my heart and the family's hearts aren't feeling a bit more fragile these days, that we'll be able to handle things at home without him, and that thirteen weeks isn't really all that long. His heaviness is the weight of everything to come. My heaviness is the weight of holding up a facade.

We've never said "goodbye"—only "I love you" when we part. Goodbye is too final, too concrete. Today is different. Even without the word spoken, it hangs in the air. I fear I'll never see him as he is right now. That if he returns, he won't be the same man who's leaving. And I don't know how to brace for that kind of change. His stride is tall, confident. His mood is somber, not unusual as he hates being away. He hesitates for one more kiss, one more hug. Going through his final checklist to make sure he has everything. "Wallet," clutching his pocket. "Phone," shows in his hand. "Charger," feels the front of his backpack. "Red Seal" feeling for the circular can of snuff in his pocket once again. "Glasses," hand to sweatshirt pocket. "Okay," he says reluctantly, "guess that's it." And it is. This is it. Today will be the first day of many when I will be repeating my silent pleas for protection.

Please protect him. Don't let him get sick. Provide him with proper equipment and seal any cracks in his immunity. Please give him mental awareness, guide his knowledge, and give him peace. Guard his soul, his spirit. Give him grace when needed for himself, space to reveal it, and calm to live with it. Shield his eyes to guard his spirit. Please, please, don't allow this to break him. Return him to us as you are taking him. Whoever is listening I beg, I plead, hear my voice. Keep him safe.

After he puts the last of his things in the truck, he turns to me, hugging me tightly. *Why do I feel like this will be the last one? Why am I forcing myself to imprint every detail about him on my soul? Why does this feel final?* I soak in every aspect of him: his smell, his breaths, the way he holds me, the way he lowers himself to my level when he feels me stretching up to him. His loving and determined eyes. His stern and oh so familiar facial lines. His tender and careful smile. His gym-callused hands that cover the length of his third, fourth and fifth fingers. His tanned skin, a reminder of our beach days.

"I love you," he breaks the silence, interrupting my assessment.

"I am so proud of you," I return. "Please be safe," I beg.

"I will, Baby. We have too much to do, too much to live for." He climbs into the truck, settles himself, kisses me one last time—another "I love you."

I hand him a journal. He looks at me puzzled. "Use it for your thoughts. Any thoughts. You can choose to share them or not. Either way, it will be a safe place where you can be truthful in what you are feeling."

Still puzzled, offering me a little eye roll, he takes it. This is not his thing. It is more a me thing. But I ask him to appease me and to use it. I know he'll need it. He'll be away from anyone that he can talk to openly. He'll be working overnight. Communication back home is going to be more challenging. I know that he'll need somewhere safe to get his thoughts out and to work through what he is experiencing and feeling.

Trying to lift the mood. He laughs, slightly, "Thank you,

Baby. I will."

"Call me," I remind him. "Every day. Be safe. I love you."

"I will, Baby. Every day. You be safe. I love you." He closes the truck door, drives away, and I stand there watching until I can no longer see his taillights in the dark of the early morning.

We have hesitantly but courageously acknowledged the fact that for the first time in twelve years of travel nursing he won't be able to come home, nor will I be able to go visit. Nothing about this time is similar or familiar to us. Going into the unknown in more ways than one has me repeating my silent cries to the universe, hoping someone, something, is listening.

I force my way back inside and immediately head to the porch. I need the comfort of this sanctuary to help me get through these first few moments of him being gone. I sink into my captain's chair, cheeks streaked with the weeks of tears I've held inside. It's just me here. No one to pretend for. No mask to wear. Right now, there isn't anything to do but allow the tears to fall freely. In the hush, an anonymous quote that I read once comes to mind with new meaning: "And once the storm is over, you won't remember how you made it through... When you come out of the storm, you won't be the same person who walked in."

Scott left saying it was "just another assignment." I'm left reckoning with an upheaval, knowing that this is anything but. this assignment will irrevocably change us.

I sit mourning the man he is today. I don't know if he'll come home, and if he does, who he'll be when this is all over. Even though there was no "goodbye" it is exactly what we just did. I forever said goodbye to the man who just drove off. I know he will never be the same after this. I breathe in, try to settle into my chair, count to ten, and repeat the only mantra that somewhat soothes: "He's trained. He's prepared. He'll come home." And for now, that has to be enough.

> *Facebook Post: The day has come. This morning at about 0545 I sent him into the darkness to be the light for so many in need. He arrived at Elmhurst (Queens NY) about 6:30 p.m.*
>
> *Quarantine is NOTHING compared to how our family is feeling at this moment and will continue for the next 13 weeks. We will at times seem as if "nothing new here" full of optimism and other days we won't be able to stop our minds from going to the darkest places. Please be patient with us. Please do not judge the smiles, laughter, and feel-good times when you think we should be full of worry and*

tearful. I can assure you that burden is part of us now even if we don't show it outwardly in every moment. We will cope the best we can.

Scott Maiers, I want you to know, you are our heartbeat. We are more than proud of the sacrifice you are about to make for others. We love you... more. Stay safe and go do what we all know you can. We are with you. We will be waiting.

CHAPTER 5

New York Arrival

I scroll through the news sites and feel the weight of the words settling in my chest. Without even seeking it out, I see information about Elmhurst. Elmhurst Hospital, dubbed the epicenter of COVID, is a 545-bed public facility in Queens, New York that has been transformed into a COVID-only fortress. The news from there is so horrifying that it makes daily headlines. And even though I don't want to look, I can't turn away because that is now where my heart exists outside my chest for the next thirteen weeks.

They transferred all non-COVID patients out, dedicating every inch to this battlefront. Qns.com
A refrigerated truck outside became a grim temporary morgue—bodies waiting to be claimed. abcnews.go.com
In one dire 24-hour span, 13 people died within those walls. Qns.com

Elmhurst isn't just another hospital—it's the epicenter of an unimaginable crisis, its hallways brimming with suffering, trauma, and courage beyond measure. Queenseagle.com

Elmhurst Hospital sits in Queens, New York City—named early on as "the center of the center" of the COVID-19 crisis. (Abcnews.go.com) By March 26, the hospital had 63 ventilators on site, 54 of which were already in use to keep critically ill patients breathing. www.politico.com

Just a day later, Elmhurst's normal operating capacity— typically around 80 percent—had swelled to roughly 125 percent as every available bed filled with COVID-19 cases and makeshift ICU pods sprang up in hallways and conference rooms. www.politico.com

I push the laptop away from me. I can't read any more right now. I can't even comprehend the scale of devastation, COVID cases, the magnitude of sickness. Death. And nurses in crisis, trying to keep up with all of it. New York, specifically Elmhurst, is nothing short of a war zone. They're fighting on a front line where every breath is a battle, risking their own lives. And some are losing the battle to the very virus they've vowed to fight. Knowing that Scott has driven straight into this abyss, my heart shatters for what he'll see, for what he'll have to do, and what he'll carry back home with him.

For months I've been watching the news each day. The TV is on as soon as I wake up and it's the last sounds I hear before bed. I am scrolling through news sites all day long trying to stay on top of every piece of information. But I pay closer attention now. Now, I have a personal investment there. My own experience in nursing, in hospitals, and with everything making the news, I can visualize what he's walking into. I picture the hallways. The overcrowded ICU. The masks, the sweat, the sound of alarms that never stop. I see him there—not just as a nurse, but as my husband. My anchor. My heart. Fighting the tears becomes harder each minute. Swallowing down my fear is a constant battle. And each hour that passes that he is away, I am reminded that love doesn't make us invincible–it makes us vulnerable.

I sit in silence staring off to the distance. Unfocused. No music. No movement. I regret that first click. An informative Google search that opened the floodgates. Now I'm drowning in it. The images. The numbers. The headlines that scream like sirens. It's sci-fi, but it's not fiction. It's *real life*. Elmhurst. Ground zero. The place where the line between life and death is thinning by the hour. As much as I want to hide away from the headlines, I keep looking. What if I miss something? What if the next update is the one that changes everything? But it's killing me. The magnitude of it. The ticker rolls like Wall Street, but these aren't stocks. These are human lives. Sick people. Dying mothers, fathers, sons, daughters. People already lost. And Scott—he is *my* person. So I look. And I keep looking. I keep reading. I keep scrolling. Every day since the world exploded with the virus has been more tragic than the previous. And it's not slowing down. There are still no answers. No solutions. No protections. It is only going to get worse. I glance at the time and feel my breath catch in my throat—he's only been gone a few hours, heading straight into all this chaos.

This is the mood that Madi walks in on. She's soft-footed, careful, like she knows I'm barely holding on by a thread. She takes the seat next to me, her presence gentle but grounding, fully aware that hours before I had sent him off.

"What are you doing?" she asks, voice low, eyes scanning my face.

I hate that I've taught her to be this attuned. To read energy like a language. To feel the emotions I'm trying so hard not to emit. Trying to be casual, I shrug. "Nothing. Just scouring the web."

She doesn't buy it. She never does. "Mom, it's okay. We are going to be okay. He is going to be okay. He always is." I wonder if she believes it or if she's saying it for both of us—casting the words like a spell, hoping they'll stick. Either way, it works. Her voice, her heart, her compassion—they're a much needed balm of protection for her momma's heart.

With Madi, I often ask myself who the adult in the room really is. Today, it's her and she doesn't even realize it. She doesn't run from it either. We make plans for dinner. Write out a market list. Coordinate our work schedules like it's any other week. And for a moment, I let the heaviness go. I settle into the rhythm of mundane tasks, the comfort of routine. But it doesn't last. Guilt creeps in, quiet and cruel. Scott is on his way to a cataclysm, and I'm here debating whether or not to have steak or burgers for dinner tonight.

The house is quiet, but my heart, it's loud—a buzz of worry, guilt, pride, all tangled together. I imagine him on the road. Windows down, the air slicing through his truck, cool and clean. He'll lean into it, breathe deeply, letting it fill his lungs. He'll have the music loud. Grateful Dead will fade into the 80s—channel 33, then 8, then 5. He never lingers on one station for long. I imagine his hands tapping the wheel.

Left foot bouncing. Eyes facing determinedly forward.

I walked through the rest of the day in a fog—half-present, half-vanishing, mostly distracted by the constant news hum. I couldn't tell you who I spoke to or what I said. Just that every time someone asked how I was holding up, I lied. "I'm fine," I muttered, like a reflex. But nothing about this was fine. And as the hours dragged on, the silence around me pressed in closer with everything I couldn't bring myself to admit or say.

...

The phone rings startlingly. I'm unaccustomed to the sound of it. For the first time in years I have taken my phone off vibrate. I can't risk missing a single call from him. I sigh in gratitude and relief. It's him.

"Hey, Baby," I say in the most upbeat voice I have.

"Hi, Honey." He sounds tired. "I made it. Man, this is weird. I am in such a busy, congested area of the city but no one is on the roads, very few people on the sidewalks. Everyone is wearing masks and going out of the other's way to be as far from anyone they are passing. It's very eerie." He sounds confused, uncomfortable.

"Oh my, I bet. What about your apartment? Does it

seem like a safe area?"

"Well, it is very apparent I am going to have some culture shock. Everything is packed very close together. It's on a one-way street. The apartment is a basement apartment with bars on the windows."

"What?! Bars on the windows!" I gasp.

"Yeah, but the apartment itself is small and very nice. The landlord left Sheila and I a bottle of wine." He says unconcerned.

"Ah that is nice. Be safe. Remember Dorothy, you are not in Kansas anymore." I say jokingly.

"I will," he laughs. "I walked to the hospital, it's 1.1 miles, a 25-minute walk through Queens. So, it will be a little over two miles each day."

"How is that? The walk? Is it safe?"

"I was a little nervous at first because the only thing I know of Queens is what I've seen on TV. But after walking a few blocks that feeling went away and I just took in the sights. This is not an affluent area," he continues. "The hospital is an old building with some updates. It looks big from where I was standing, takes up about a city block. While I was there, five ambulances came and went," he says as if giving a report with no hesitation in his voice. What I hear is urgency, excited energy. I hear him wanting to get in there and do his part.

He tells me Sheila arrived around 7:30 p.m. after saying goodbye to her babies and boarding a plane from Myrtle Beach earlier that day.

Scott and Sheila will be sharing the apartment for their time at Elmhurst. Sheila flew up to New York and Scott went by her house the day before and packed all her things in the truck he was driving up. And, in true Sheila-style, it wasn't just her necessities that she packed. It was totes upon totes full of anything and everything they could possibly need for their time there.

Toilet paper, paper towels, sanitizer, cleaning supplies, Scentsy smell goods—every possible comfort and contingency. She thought of everything. That's who she is. She knew they wouldn't have time to think once they got there. She prepared for store shelves being bare, and exhaustion being constant. Scott, on the other hand, had a couple of bags and one tote. That's who he is. Minimalist. Driven. Pack light, move fast, save the world. Thanks to her, he'd have everything he didn't think to bring. Everything he didn't know he'd need. It was love, packed in plastic bins. Preparedness wrapped in lavender-scented wax melts. A friendship confirmation to us both that said, I've got you, even when the world was falling apart.

"Did you get your first day instructions yet?" I ask.

"No," he says, frustrated. "I will have to email my recruiter and hospital manager in the morning."

After asking him to get some rest I remind him about his journal, hoping that he'll use it. "I won't forget," he said. "I am going to write before I go to sleep."

"Okay, Baby, I love you, I miss you." I say softly. I feel like I can't say it enough.

"I love you, Baby, and I miss you so much," he says.

Ending the call is so hard and it's only day one.

It's only thirteen weeks, I think to myself trying to talk myself through it. *I can do anything for thirteen weeks. Just 91 days, only 2,184 hours which is 131,040 minutes.* Doing the rapid calculations trying to figure out which number sounds shortest to make it potentially easier to accept. Now, I sit and breathe deep and make a plan to attempt to force the next 13 weeks/91 days/2,184 hours/131,040 minutes to go by quickly.

Work will be a distraction. I commit myself to being the best clinical manager I can. The drive to and from work will take up four hours of my day. I'll find a book or a podcast to listen to so I'm not hearing the news for hours a day. He will call every day. We'll text as often as possible. I'll journal too. I'll need somewhere to let it all out—a place where I don't have to be guarded and no filter. That's how I'll get through each day. One page at a time.. Maybe I'll even blog about it. Madi and I will plan to workout at the house, cook together, and just hang out.

Spending time with her is a silver lining in all this. This seems like a good plan. A focused, intentional distraction so that I can keep myself together and be strong for all of us. But the hard truth is that I have zero motivation to do any of it. I just want to crawl into bed and ignore everything until he's safe and home again.

Damn, this is going to be a long 13 weeks, 91 days, 2,184 hours, 131,040 minutes, my heart voice whispers.

CHAPTER 6

First Impressions

DAY 1- ELMHURST HOSPITAL, APRIL 14, 2020.

W e didn't get first day instructions, so Sheila and I just went over to the hospital at 0800," he tells me, disgustedly.

"That's irritating and odd. You have never not gotten instructions. How did you know where to go?" I asked.

"He continues on like he didn't hear my questions. "There was no one out when we walked to the hospital. Remember when we came for Christmas Eve and how busy it was? Remember we kept bumping into people, all the lines to get on the subway. There is none of that. There is no one out on the street. It's eerie. The city that never sleeps... It's deserted, a ghost town practically."

I'm trying to picture it and I can't. We were there for Christmas a few years ago. It was insane how many people were there. We expected it to some extent, of course, it's New York City at Christmas, but even still. It was so much more than we planned for. So trying to imagine what the city looks like without all of that hustle and vibrancy, is difficult.

"When we got to the hospital, several buses, like the buses people go on trips in, fucking charter buses, full of Krucial Rapid Response nurses were parked outside. Must be really short staffed here in order to bring travel nurses like us and then also have Krucial nurses here. "

My heart sinks. Krucial nurses! Krucial Rapid Response nurses are only brought in when there is a crisis—catastrophies. They're contracted to work twenty-one days straight for twelve-hour days, then re-contracted for another twenty-one days if needed, with only a few days off in between contracts. Even knowing that Krucial nurses have been contracted and that they are only brought in under the most dire circumstances, Scott's voice doesn't change. He isn't shocked. There is no hesitancy. No crack to his voice. Just calm, steady. As always. His agenda remains the same: Save the world.

"So they direct us to an auditorium, telling us we will get directions there."

"How many of you were there to start today?" I ask.

"The auditorium was full. But what was really crazy..." he continues. "As we are walking to it there are a lot of people dressed in fatigues."

"Fatigues? For what? Security?"

"No, they are Army, Navy, and Air Force, all of them nurses, docs, respiratory therapists."

My heart voice is on alert by now. This is not normal. This is not like a Chicken Little warning, "The sky is falling!" It already has, and my husband and my best friend are running head first into it. Armageddon, I don't know what that would look or feel like, I don't know if it even is a thing, but my heart voice is telling me, *We are here. This is it.*

"We were only in the auditorium for a couple of hours, kinda an overview of what we might see, PPE requirements, and statistics they had so far. They said 150 patients on vents running currently, all COVID positive. One of the first people I met was the assistant manager of the ED at MUSC. [Emergency department at Medical University of South Carolina] He told me he had been one of the 900 laid off." He chuckles. "Really makes me wonder what the fuck is going on. Nurses being laid off as hospitals should be getting ready to gear up for the shit I saw today."

"Wow, laying off people is so, crazy. So, in your past

experience, how many vents have you seen run at once?" I ask, really not wanting to know the answer.

He's quiet a moment before he answers, "Twenty is a lot, twenty is a high number for a place like this. Now if you go to a place like University of Maryland you could see more. I'd say that in a hospital of this size they probably only have twenty-five. They told us because of the amount needed they have a bunch of different types and company loaners along with transport vents."

"Transport vents?"

"Yeah, but those cannot be used for long periods of time so not sure how that is working," he replies definitively.

"They have PPE?"

"Yeah, they told us they had plenty. They said that they received donations because they were one of the hardest hit hospitals."

"How many COVID units?"

"The entire hospital is now a COVID unit. They are turning everything else away, only intakes are COVID patients. The entire hospital is a COVID ICU."

He still isn't shaken. Still determined. Still focused on one thing. He is undeterred by what he learned today.

"I am going to SAVE as many as I can." ...or die trying,

my heart voice adds. "After we were done there, they took us up to CCU. [Cardiac Care Unit].The unit itself is typical, clean. Looked to be well stocked. I am paired with a really cool nurse, Alvin. He goes by, Al. He tells me that they have lost so many and not only patients but their own staff. He said that so many employees, nurses, docs, techs, all got sick before they knew what it was. Al says all this while showing me the six full rooms they are using to store the belongings of the patients who have died."

Oh my god, this is why so many additional Krucial and travel nurses have been brought in. Staffing is short because their own have died or are sick and unable to work, on top of the rapid number of patients coming in and not getting any better.

"The unit is 10-12 beds. Every bed is full. It is like walking into a hazmat scene. People of all ages. A 27 year old just died. There are two 30 year old guys here, vented, no past medical history. No family allowed to visit. Everyone in the unit is on a vent. Alvin and I had two patients tonight, but he told me that the week before we got there it was common to have seven patients per nurse."

"SEVEN!!!" The word ripped out of me like a warning shot. In ordinary times—without a novel virus choking every unit—three patients per nurse is already pushing the edge of safe care. But seven? That's not just overwhelming. That's dangerous. That's a battlefield.

"He is beyond grateful for all of us coming." Scott must hear the terror and concern in my voice so he reminds me, "Baby, this is why I came."

I could not argue that. I feel so much pride in him for the choice he made to be someone willing to jump in and help when things are this bad.

He continues. "People are really sick, and you can see the nurses are tired. I see it in their eyes, through their steamed-up shields or goggles, or both for some. Many haven't had any days off. I am gonna have to figure something out for my head though."

"What do you mean, something for your head?"

"Because the masks are tearing my head up, it's so sore and it's only been one day." He sighs. "When you enter the hospital, you have to have a mask on, like a normal surgical mask. They told us during auditorium orientation that all patient care areas were Level 3. I've heard of air borne precautions, contact, droplet, and neutropenic precautions. I've never heard of a Level 3. Which basically means hazmat suit, but we don't have them so when we get off the elevator to our unit, all the doors are shut, every single door, patient rooms, shut; unit entrance, shut; literally every hospital door, shut. We have to go to the break room to put our personal stuff down. All the things we typically hide at our stations on the unit, we couldn't take in, including our stethoscope, they have disposable ones we have to use. We could take our own pen or scissors but not much else, no drinks or snacks. From there we went to antepartum room, where we get all our PPE—green paper scrubs put directly over the scrubs we're wearing, pull on shoe covers that came to our knees, with a blue plastic gown on top of that, N95 with surgical mask over it, shield or goggles over eyes. Baby, I need goggles, I can't do the shield."

"Okay I will order on Amazon right now and send them to you." The Amazon cart is being loaded with purpose, in real time.

"We have to wear the thin little net cap thing. You know the ones they put on you before surgery, well we had to wear them. I need to get some thicker surgical caps because my head is raw from those thin little caps and the mask straps rubbing."

"Okay, I will get you both some of them." This feels good. I can channel my fear and feelings of uselessness into action. This can be my mission. I will contact Momma Jo and get her in on this, then maybe we both can feel like we are doing something.

"After all that layering is done, we put gloves on and enter the actual unit for assignment. Everywhere you see Level 3 in big black letters on fire engine red signs, plastered all over the walls. It is so hot with all the layers of PPE. So get this, I forgot to tell ya..."

"What?" Do I even want to hear this? Can I handle hearing it?

"We were told we had to reuse our N95 masks. None of us were fit tested there, I am not sure if others were done prior to getting here but honestly, it doesn't matter. When we got to the PPE room there was a hodge podge of N95s stacked haphazardly on the shelves. We had to pick which we thought would be best fit, for me I knew which I had used previously so I was lucky today to be able to find the style I've used before—the duck bill one is the one that fits me, the green ones you use don't fit me. After our shift when we take it all off, we are told to put it in the paper bag, put our names on it and leave it in the PPE room for our next shift and the next four shifts."

"Reuse N95!?!" My mind is whirling. Are you kidding

me?! A paper bag! A week using the same N95 mask! Where the fuck is JCAHCO and all their medical standards now?

JCAHCO, what a joke, my mind huffs. They can come in and ding you for having a drink at the nurses' station or any minor thing like that, but now, during a pandemic, they're nowhere to be found. Infection control is the reason for their existence. COVID is the gasoline being poured onto a wildfire, one that isn't even close to being contained. It's getting stronger, hotter, and burning, not through acres but through human lives. Yet, where is JCAHCO in all this? Are they cowardly hiding in their safe space? I don't know, maybe in their private hazmat suite, while my husband must trust his triple layer of paper/plastic scrubs? Are they breathing purified air while my husband inhales his own breath? Are they surrounded by their family, while I sit here six hundred and seventy-seven miles away from mine, desperately waiting for every ring of my phone just to hear his voice? Are they having long chats over coffee with their loved ones while there are patients having to say their final goodbyes through a video call organized by a stranger only for their families on the other side of the phone to see them connected to machines just barely keeping them alive for a few moments more. Are they sipping on fruity drinks pool side, while my husband hasn't even tasted water in twelve hours?

Ever since nursing school and all the years of being a nurse, we have always been told that N95s are one time use, per JCAHCO standard. And now in the middle of a pandemic it's all of sudden okay to go ahead and re-use...?? I despise the government departments today. This is personal, my husband is running headfirst into this and has taken the personal risk to save us all. He chose this voluntarily from the purest servant heart. Now, during a declared pandemic, one of the biggest accreditation bodies of medical care could care less for their own standards and are nowhere to be found.

In my rage I head to the JCAHCO website. And right there is their mission statement:

"The mission of Joint Commission is to continuously improve health care for the public, in collaboration with other stakeholders, by evaluating health care organizations and inspiring them to excel in providing safe and effective care of the highest quality and value." Jointcommision.org

Laughable is my first thought. Anger is second. *Continuously improve health care for the public.* Seriously? By reusing an N95 that is in the COVID abyss? *Along with stakeholders...* Okay there it is, how many "stakeholders" are on the frontlines at this very minute? *...inspiring...* Not even close, you want inspiring, I can single-handedly give you inspiring in the flesh and blood, his name is Scott Maiers, RN. I refuse for him to be their sacrificial lamb. My blood is boiling.

Mental note: Best to stay off the web for my own sanity.

"Baby, Baby? You still there?"

Startled out of my own fuming thoughts. "Yes, I am still here."

"Why are you so quiet," he asks

What I wanted to tell him was that I am so scared for him and us. What I said instead was, "No reason, just can't believe you have to re-use an N95!"

"I know," he says, "it's crazy. I was always told single-use." He continues, "Then all this gear we have to wear. It is so hot. I'm sweating before I even get report for my shift. But I guess I better try and get some sleep, tomorrow night I am in my unit. On my own, they call it 'Tour 1.' Orientation is complete." He pauses for a few breaths and then tells me, "I miss you so much. This is going to be a long thirteen weeks."

That is the first time he has acknowledged that.

"I am going to try and get some kind of workout in here at the apartment before work."

"Okay, but please make sure you don't push yourself. You will need as much sleep and rest as you can get. Sounds like some grueling days ahead. Don't forget to write in your journal."

"I won't. I do it before I go to bed. I'll be fine, don't worry about me. Make sure you and the kids are listening to the guidelines and staying in and wearing your mask everywhere. I don't know what I would do if something happened to you or the kids." Still unshaken. Not only attempting to save everyone at Elmhurst, but all of us back home too.

And just like every other time we get off the phone since we've been apart, I begin my silent prayers. *Dear universe please, please protect him physically. Wrap your arms around his heart and shield his eyes from sights no human should witness. Bring him home to me and the kids.*

I worry about when he's going to break. I worry about him getting sick. I am overwhelmed by the fear of those worries becoming reality. He is ass-deep in COVID for forty-eight hours a week for the next thirteen weeks with an N95 that has to be reused for an entire week. I know him. He is and will continue to take every precaution. He will hate every minute of it but will do it. He understands the COVID risk. He understands the physical health risks, even if he doesn't yet understand the risk to his spirit. But I do. So I sit here, alone, wondering how long it will take before his heart voice begins to scream.

After I hang up, I don't cry. I click. I search. I add everything he needs to the Amazon cart. Goggles. Thicker skull caps. Barrier cream. Skin prep. Anything to ease the wounds left behind from the straps of the masks and the metal bar that grips the bridge of his nose. I imagine him peeling off the mask after twelve hours, his skin raw, his breath stale, his spirit fraying. So I built a fortress for him in my Amazon cart. One item at a time. Then I message Momma Jo. I tell her about the headbands I saw on Facebook—the ones with buttons sewn near the ears so the surgical mask loops don't dig into the skin. She replies instantly: "Don't worry, Baby. I've got this." She's already thinking bigger. She'll gather her friends. They'll sew, stitch, and deliver. Not just for Scott and BFF, but for anyone who needs them. We're building something now. A quiet rebellion against the ache. A resistance made of fabric and thread.

CHAPTER 7

Tour One

QUEENS, NY: APRIL 15, 2020 - DAY 2

Waking and still a little groggy he gets up. Takes his phone and starts scrolling. Coffee being brewed. Steak and eggs being prepped for *dinner*. Ketones mixed for the mile walk to work. BFF is up and immediately gets on her phone, checking on the kids, hubby, ma. They sit and eat scrambled eggs and bacon for *breakfast*. Night shifters eat *dinner* at 0300 and *breakfast* at 1600. Conversation between them is small talk, weather, what they're packing for lunch tonight, time they should leave to ensure arrival allows for the time to put on all the layers of gear.

Both are awestruck by how empty the streets are. Not your typical vision of NYC, full of life, hustling and bustling at all hours. Horns blaring, whistles blowing, sirens, the constant clapping of shoes against the pavement, conversations overlapping and weaving in and out as millions of people go about their days. It's all been replaced by the ever-present rhythmic sound of the sirens echoing from every direction reminding them of the task at hand.

"Did they tell you about the staff here?" BFF asks.

"Yeah, crazy. Staying in hotels for fear of taking it home to their families," Scott says matter-of-factly, unscathed by it.

"What do you think about the two minute code time? Like who is really doing that?" she asks.

In non-medical terms, a Code Blue means someone's dying—and fast. Normally, the team doesn't stop trying to save them for twenty, sometimes thirty minutes. But here, they were told they only had two minutes.

"Yeah, this is crazy shit. I can tell you this, I won't be doing that, they will have to physically drag me out. No way can we determine effectiveness in two fucking minutes," he tells her.

"Yeah, me either," she agrees.

Approaching the hospital they both notice their insides doing a dance, neither acknowledge it nor speak of it. They remember being told there weren't enough oxygen tanks so people have to sit in circles, gathered around an oxygen tank spliced off to nasal cannulas and masks all sharing the same tank.

They spend the rest of the walk into the hospital talking through all the instructions and information they got during their overly quick orientation the day before. The entire hospital is a Level 3 Zone, meaning full PPE required the entire time in patient care areas. *152 vents running... two minute code time... complete lack of resources...* They both feel the undeniable anxiety of what they're facing and yet they still can't quite comprehend it really being as bad as they say. It's been over thirty days since the U.S. declared a pandemic. It still feels surreal. Scott, however, with a confidence born from twenty years of nursing isn't scared for himself; he only questions how they're going to be able to handle so many patients who are so incredibly sick. He thinks nothing more than that this is going to be just a little busier than usual.

Walking into the hospital they hear something familiar. Both their hearts drop. Blaring over the loud speaker is Alicia Keys and Jay Z singing about their love of New York.

In New York,
Concrete jungle where dreams are made of
There's nothing you can't do
Now you're in New York

These streets will make you feel brand new
The lights will inspire you
Lets hear it for New York
New York, New York

This song will never be heard in the same spirit for either of them.

They pass by the area where various businesses have so graciously provided a bagged lunch for the staff. Scott won't eat most of it. He is diligent about what he puts in his body. Not because he watches the scale or is concerned with his appearance, but because he believes that what we put into our bodies directly impacts the response or prevention of disease our bodies are able to have. His theory is certainly going to be put to the test these upcoming weeks. And yes, he is disciplined, this is also about him exerting a sense of control in a situation that feels very much out of control.

Regardless, he takes the bag, looks inside, sees the sandwich and cookie and/or chips provided and puts it in his backpack knowing he will give it away to a fellow nurse or the homeless guy they often encounter on their walk to and from the hospital.

They navigate their way to the unit. The designated path through the hospital is unusual. Under normal circumstances, staff would be able to enter the unit and walk around freely without restriction. This is very different. They have to enter the unit from a specified location, walk on marked hallways to reach certain rooms. Everything is routed and clearly mapped out. Roaming is not allowed.

The first stop on the route through the unit is where he will leave his backpack and retrieve his brown bag with his N95 for the week. He forces the mask over his head. Since this wasn't specifically fitted for him, the straps are too tight and when he molds the metal nose piece snug, he winces. He exaggerates his breaths in and out checking for leaks. None, so he moves on to the next stop.

Here he retrieves his plastic scrubs that go over his Jockey scrubs, then his gown that goes over his plastic scrubs that are over his Jockey scrubs. Then his shoe covers, which go over his shoes, over the plastic scrubs, that are over the Jockey scrubs. Goggles on over the N95, adjusting the straps of both the goggles and mask flinching slightly, his head is already sore and irritated from the straps. He's already sweating because of all the layers. Next come the gloves. He searches for the correct size wondering how the hell he is supposed to put the damn gloves on sweaty hands. And he's not even inside the unit yet where the work begins.

He gets the gloves on, heads toward the unit, taps his badge on the door, and walks in. It's the first day inside the unit where he will spend the next thirteen weeks.

Alarms welcome his arrival. Everyone is running. The nurse to the left is calling a code. He sees Alvin, one of the few staff RNs, who greets him with smiling eyes and says "Welcome" in a beaten-down voice.

4/11/20: United States: 20,071 deaths; 522,000 confirmed cases. New York reports 783 new cases with 8600 deaths.

What he encounters in his unit plays like an end-of-days movie. So many young people are so sick. A twenty-four year old female, Fancy's age, oxygen saturation 85-88% on high ventilator settings, in kidney failure with ARDS (acute respiratory distress).

CODE BLUE pierces across the unit, he runs.

Oxygen levels are rapidly dropping during an attempted extubation. Nothing is stabilizing them. Without hesitation, Scott barges into the room, grabs ambu mask, and starts bagging. With every squeeze of that bag, he manually forces much needed oxygen into his patient's lungs, yelling, "Someone call the doctor! He needs to reintubate." Looking up to see who is following his demands, he sees five to six nurses on the outside, yelling back at him through the glass,

"Get out!" "You can't do that!" "We aren't allowed to do that." Their screams, for Scott's safety, are begging him to get out of the room. Their muffled pleas, the wide eyes pressed close to glass separating them from him, remind him that bagging a COVID positive patient intensifies the spread of the virus by forcing contaminated air in your air. And still, Scott doesn't stop.

He yells out what he is seeing on the monitors. "Bipap settings 24/12, O2 sats are in the 70s on 100% O2."

"I am NOT going to stand here doing nothing. Get the damn doctor now!" he demands.

"You can't, the virus, the aerosol," they beg.

"I don't care, I am here to save lives. I am not leaving! Call the damn doctor now!!!"

A doctor arrives telling Scott to, "Go ahead and go, we've got it from here," while checking his own mask, and getting his stuff together.

"I am not leaving, get your stuff ready, I'm bagging him until you are ready," Scott responds through clenched teeth, pronouncing each word with command.

Their eyes meet, they both realize in this battle neither

are leaving, both with the same goal. In this gaze, the profound mutual respect to each other not only as colleagues, but warriors, unspoken but understood. This was one of the Navy doctors deployed. Dr Kochan turns, grabs the intubation kit. Hearing the 'click' he knows the scope is together.

"Ready?" Scott asks, looking at Dr. Kochan.

"Suction," followed by gentle, quick movements as his hands guide the scope down the throat, "I'm in," Dr. Kochan continues, with each step spoken aloud.

"Cuff is inflated," Scott responds.

Dr. Kochan, in constructive collaboration, checks the chest for breaths. "Adjust the settings," Dr. Kochan instructs. "That's as good as it can be, 89%."

Chest x-ray obtained for placement. It's confirmed, placement is good.

"Okay, breathe," Scott softly encourages his patient, subconsciously giving himself the same encouragement.

"SHIT!! He's dropping!! CODE BLUE!" Scott yells. Two more doctors and two more nurses come running.

Scott jumps up on the gurney and begins chest compressions. "1,2,3,4,.." he counts aloud, pushing deep into his patient's chest, sweat beading on his skin, bleeding through his cap under the straps, goggles fogging from the heat coming off his skin. "1,2,3,4,5,6,..." he continues, the snaps of ribs breaking beneath his hands, expected but still he cringes as he feels them snap. The other nurses, chaotic to the naked eye, are pulling medications, the sound of the medication syringe caps falling to the tiled floor, the doctors are calling out orders for medications.

"Meds in," one nurse interjects.

"1,2,3,4,5,6,7,.."

No one is saying it out loud but everyone is feeling the same cry within: "NOTHING IS WORKING! WHY IS NOTHING WORKING?!"

Time of Death: 2200.

Nurses begin gathering up the debris, it's robotic, auto-pilot. Task oriented. Trash, red bag, needle container, retrieval of the body bag. Dr. Kochan stops and speaks, "Let's take a minute. This man died without his family, let's be that for him."

Deafening silence.

Scott feels the heat and sting of his eyes. *DAMN IT!!* The thought is angry. *He was only two years older than me.* Consumed by these thoughts, he starts to pull off what's left of the blue plastic gown—torn, ripped, and sweat-stuck to him—it's turned into paper-mâché.

No preexisting conditions! He had a wife, kids. Scott's rage is escalating, his heart is racing, and he is still trying to break the adhesion of the plastic gown from his skin. *What is wrong with these things? They are so wet they won't come off!* Mumbling what he thinks is under his breath. Looks up to see the others watching him just as the blue plastic gown breaks free from his body

"I need a minute to dry off, I'll be back."

Leaving the room, he looks down at what's left. His body is hugged tightly in sweat-saturated layers. The green paper scrubs are adhered to his normal everyday navy scrubs. He notices the sting from the bridge of his nose, his cheeks, ears, and the top of his head as the salty sweat merges with his irritated and now raw skin. The friction of straps upon straps to hold his cap in place along with both his masks are pulled tightly across his face and head. His breath is dry and hot every time he breathes it back in. The echo of the door closing behind him shakes him.

He rapid-fire questions what happened in that room. *What just happened? What did we miss? Did I do everything? I should have bagged more, harder. I should have gone in sooner. Why did nothing help? I have taken care of these things before, some didn't make it but we could always give rationale to the why.*

Nothing worked for him, no preexisting conditions, he came in on a fucking nasal cannula, some shortness of breath, three days ago, by day two he was on a BiPap titrating up, day three he seemed to be doing better. This is FUCKING DAY 4! WHAT THE HELL!! What are we doing? What are we not doing? What is this? What is happening?

CODE BLUE! He rips off the green paper scrubs, snatches another set, quickly redresses, covering himself with another blue plastic gown and runs toward the alarm.

Hours turn into days, days into weeks. CODE BLUEs continue to be called. Cases of COVID continue to climb. Body bags continue to be zipped.

4/18/20: NY reports 2000 hospital admissions in the past 24 hours.

A fifty-two year old male is not doing well this morning. He was extubated on a BiPap machine that helps people breathe when they're struggling to do it on their own. It uses a mask to gently push air into the lungs—giving more pressure when you breathe in, and less when you breathe out. That makes breathing easier and keeps your airways open, especially during sleep. He is still unresponsive and is working hard to breathe even with the help of BiPap. His BiPap settings are at the highest and his oxygen levels continue to drop. Scott has to call the family. The call connects, frantic voices blare in his ear, "Do everything. Re-intubate him." He knows he would feel and say the same thing if it were his own family. That plea—so familiar, so human—echoes in his chest. But his clinical brain analyzes the data, the trajectory, the futility. It's the collision of compassion and reality that drains him. These calls don't just exhaust him because of what he has to say—they exhaust him because of what he must feel when doing it and keep going anyway.

That's the cruel fracture of COVID. Families weren't allowed in. They couldn't witness the quick unraveling. Many of these patients arrived at Elmhurst awake, talking—short of breath and requiring oxygen, maybe febrile, maybe coughing—but still themselves. That's how their families left them. Hours later, Scott is the one telling them their loved one is dying.

Despite doing everything they never were able to get his oxygen levels to recover. This sweet patient endured a needle decompression to his chest for a small pneumothorax, he underwent ultrasounds looking for everything, hoping for something that could help. He coded twice, Scott worked for him, with him, on him, for over three hours. He held his hand as he died so he would not be alone.

Looking at his watch. He is tired. The same serenade of sirens and alarms that greet him at night as he begins his shift are the same ones that send him home each morning. He is living like the *Groundhog Day* movie. Each day the same, trying over and over again to make a difference in the outcome. It's been two weeks and every shift is the same or worse.

He's exhausted. Mentally. Physically. Spiritually. Emotionally. He leaves the hospital each night hoping for any amount of sleep that he can get. Tonight, as he walks out of his unit he hears "CODE BLUE" over the intercom. Another tragedy. Another life. Another family left grieving.

He has only been gone for roughly ten hours when he walks back into his unit to start another shift. There is a forty-eight year old male who was brought into the hospital two days ago. He is a father of two sons. COVID positive. He has had a rapid advancement of ARDS in two days. He is at the highest settings for ventilation. During the first rounds, his urine output tells Scott that he is close to kidney failure and will be needing dialysis. Morning labs aren't back yet, but he knows what they will say. He's seen it over and over, day after day, now for two weeks. It goes downhill fast from here. All he can do is make sure this patient, who is more to him than simply a patient, is as comfortable as possible. He cleans his face gently. Scott's heart feels another fissure. He knows this man will never see his sons again, and his sons will never see their dad again. He feels the heaviness of his own Dad-heart thinking about Garrett, Jordan, and Zach, his own sons.

This man is not the first, and Scott knows he won't be the last. There was the forty-two year old father who came in gasping and was gone within hours, the elderly woman who whispered her grandson's name until the BiPAP drowned it out, the twenty-four year old young girl whose lungs collapsed knowing her mother wouldn't arrive– visitors of any kind– even a mother couldn't be with her child. Each one chips away pieces of him. The pace is relentless, the grief cumulative. He doesn't just carry their stories; he absorbs their final moments, their unfinished goodbyes. It's a quiet kind of devastation, the kind that settles deep into the marrow and doesn't relinquish its hold.

Another twelve hour shift is over. As he begins the long process of getting ready to leave for the day, he wonders if these nights will get any better soon. It takes twenty-five minutes to peel off the sweat-soaked, plastic-wrapped armor of PPE. Each layer clings like a magnet. His skin burns, his body aches, his spirit worn. Exhausted and drained, he reaches for the brown paper bag, gently tucks his tethered mask inside, and grabs the complimentary meal—one small gesture in a day full of chaos. He'll pass it to his homeless friend on the way home, hoping that act of kindness might offer some balm to a soul worn thin by too much loss, too many hours, and too few answers.

He snaps a quick selfie—not for vanity, but for evidence. He wants a closer look at the damage: the raw grooves across his nose, the sting along his cheeks, the soreness etched into his scalp. He gently places the tethered N95 mask back into the bag, careful not to damage it further. It has to last two more shifts. The next one begins in less than twelve hours. He reaches for the "happy" mask. The one with the colorful dancing bears that he wears outside of the hospital. A rebellion or placebo to his spirit. A flicker of hope. He pulls it on, hoping their energy might seep into his skin, hoping the morning air will fill his lungs, hoping something—*anything*—might help cleanse the ugliness seared into his soul. He glances in the mirror. His eyes are tired, dark, hollow, staring blankly back at him. His face is worn.

His posture is slumped in defeat—broken by the shift he

just finished. The morning air hits his lungs, cool and clean, a stark contrast to the recycled air of the ICU. He takes it in slowly. His walk back to the apartment begins with heavy steps, each one echoing the cadence of his spirit. He's still trying to process the night. His breaths start coming faster. His pace quickens. There's an urgency to move. He's not sure why. Maybe it's adrenaline. Maybe it's an attempted escape from his nightly reality with no end in sight—the endless loop of alarms, gasping breaths, and final goodbyes that cling to him long after he's scrubbed out. The apartment offers no true refuge, just a quieter space to replay the chaos. He walks faster, as if outrunning the weight of the lives lost, the ones slipping through his fingers despite every effort. But the grief follows. It always does.

He finds gratitude that most people aren't witnessing what he sees every night. The eyes that grow big and wide when breathing is no longer natural and they're suffocating. Blackened toes, fingers, and scrotums from spontaneous blood clots. Lips in hues of purple and blues from low oxygen levels. Tubes of all sizes in every orifice, one for urine, one for poop, one for secretions, one for fluid collecting in the chest. Eyes taped shut to protect them from drying out. No one should have to witness this. Each shift adds weight.

Another night of relentless alarms, each one a jolt to the nervous system. Another moment where he holds a hand that will soon go cold. It's not just one thing. Its all of it. Layered. Tragedies and heartache and despair stacked one on top of the other. Wearing down the edges of his spirit, piece by piece. He tells himself he's fine. He has to be. But the cracks are forming—quiet, invisible, persistent.

CHAPTER 8

The Day It Broke Him

(JOURNAL ENTRY: APRIL 21, 2020) – *It's raining, most times rain brings such a peace knowing Mother Nature's way of nourishing her Earth. I think of it often as a cleansing, calm and peaceful. But the rain now is the literal way of describing my insides. Dreary, air is heavy and stagnant, raindrops depict my soul's tears; no cleansing but rather sadness spilling from inside me. Starting slow and steady, moving too fast, aggressive; thunder is my soul yelling and the lightning are flashes that allows me full view of what is in front, around me.*

APRIL 21, 2020 MYRTLE BEACH SC

The beauty of another day is that it makes us one day closer to him returning to us. The sadness is it's only one day closer—we still have eighty days to go. Already I feel as if I'm walking through the motions of life, just like Scott, my days feel like *Groundhog Day*. On the outside, I force the appearance of being fine, that everything is as okay as it can be, and that we're all managing. On the inside, it's turmoil. The only thing I can focus on is when he is going to call and wondering what he is doing. I play a game with myself, looking at the clock, seeing the time, and imagining what he's doing. It's silly, I know, but it helps me feel closer to him. It helps me feel like we're together in this even though we're hundreds of miles apart.

Well it's 0900, he is sleeping.

It's 1200, I know he is up by now, has probably already eaten breakfast, his typical eggs and bacon, has had his coffee, ketones. He has checked his email, probably cleared them out and then raged through Facebook. I wish he would either unfriend people or not go into that space.

He is now probably trying to figure out what he can do to pass time, a walk to the store or around town maybe.

My phone vibrates on my desk, startling me out of my own head. It's a good morning text from him. I love these. After a few easy messages about our days are sent back and forth, the little text bubble appears, disappears, and reappears.

Scott: I am gonna send a few pics of my face and head. Want your opinion on what you think may help.

He sends three pictures.

The first two pictures are a left and right profile then a forward profile view. The first thing I notice are his eyes. I see the pain they expose, the depths of what they have seen. They're dark and hollow, reflecting the horrors from each night at the hospital. These experiences have been branded into him, just as I feared they would. There was no escaping it, though. I notice the rest of his face next. He's not smiling, there is no silly face like he would ordinarily make when sending me a photo. His cheeks are red and raw with indentations from the constant mask straps being worn for hours, night after night.

I leave my desk and walk outside. I need some air to process what I'm seeing. I can't help but ask if he's okay. I see that he's not, so I don't know why I'm asking. Of course, though, he says he's fine.

Scott: What about my head and cheeks, you think if I use skin prep that would help?

Jodi: Skin prep, yeah...

I text back distractedly as I continue to look closely at the photos he sent. He looks terrible. He says he's fine, but I try again.

Jodi: Honey, are you alright?

Scott: I am fine! Why do you continue to ask me that?!

I wonder if he's even looked at these pictures he sent me. If he had, he would know why I was asking. I don't say anything, though. I wonder if his denial of his current state is a coping mechanism, knowing he still has a number of weeks left of this hell.

The text bubbles continue for what seems like ten minutes, playing hide-and-seek, now you see me, now you don't. Appearing. Disappearing. Until finally... a series of texts come through.

Scott: I mean, I am tired, I am exhausted, I am sick of hearing about COVID, I am sick of spending four nights in hell. I am sick that every conversation I have with anyone is about COVID, wanting my thoughts, wanting to know what I am seeing. NO ONE wants to hear the truth of WHAT I AM SEEING.

Scott: What I see goes something like this: People on

a ventilator and people die! If we are lucky, we get 45 mins between one death and the call of another one that needs intubated and ICU. They don't stop coming. We are not seeing many stay extubated and get better.

Scott: I am sorry baby, I don't mean to take this out on you.

Scott: So many people reach out to me thanking me and calling me a hero.

I can sense him shaking his head as he's typing this.

Scott: Hero, really! I am no hero with the way things are going. I am holding hands and talking to them just so they know somehow they are not alone.

Scott: Talking to you and the kids keeps me going and I can't wait to get home to you all. I love you and gotta go get ready for another night of hell. I'll call you on my walk in. I love you.

Me and my unsettled spirit return to my desk and slump down in my chair. His pictures continue to flash before my eyes, tattooed to the back of my lids. I can't unsee his eyes. I feel their pain. If it is true that our spirit reveals itself through our eyes, his spirit has broken, no longer strong enough to avoid the inevitable shatter, no longer able to deny the overwhelming feeling of defeat. No more silent strength. No more borrowed hope. Just the raw, unfiltered truth of a man who has given everything and watched it slip away. Today is the day. The day it broke him. Not in a loud, dramatic collapse—but in the quiet, soul-crushing way that leaves no visible wound yet bleeds from the inside out. The day his body finally listened, while his heart whispers, "How much more?"

I look around me. The desk I sit at each day. The minimal staff in the office now. Everyone keeping their distance, afraid to come within six feet of each other. Masks covering half of their faces. The phone that my nurses use asking me to bring them things to avoid entry in the building. They're following instructions to protect us. Me? Them? Who exactly is being protected from this? I have an employee, a hospice aide, currently in the hospital who is intubated right alongside her mother. She is the sole provider, both monetarily and personally, for her family. She has children. They certainly haven't been protected from anything.

I continue to look with blank eyes around the office. I see the colorful flyer advertising the food drive for her family. The locked cabinet that contains the three masks per employee I am instructed by my boss to tally, track, and divvy out accordingly. "Only three Jodi, they will get three new ones each week." Apparently somewhere along the lines the 'brown paper bag method' has been determined as safe.

What are you doing Jodi? My heart voice questions. *All of this is against every fiber of your soul. Scott is on the frontlines, giving everything for his colleagues and patients while you sit in your "ivory tower" protected. This is not what you want to be doing.*

Then I remember Scott's words. "Baby you stay here. One of us needs to be safe and here for the kids." His words stay with me but they don't quiet my heart voice that is getting more persistent as the days pass. A call is churning within me. I have to do something more than what I am doing.

CHAPTER 9

Answering My Call

Sitting down at my desk, I pull out my phone and text a clinical manager from one of my previous nursing assignments.

Jodi: Darlene, it's Jodi, hope all is well there. I wanted to see if you have any needs for a travel nurse.

I see a response coming immediately.

Darlene: Jodi, it is so good to hear from you. Let me check with HR. I know we do need help. These are crazy times. We have nurses out sick and patients coming on faster than we can keep up with. Give me about an hour and I'll get back to you.

I worked with Darlene as my clinical manager for my very first hospice travel nurse contract at Duke University. It was the best first assignment for a newbie. I extended my first contract there, staying for an additional four weeks, and kept an ongoing friendship with her after I left.

Less than twenty minutes go by and my phone vibrates. It's a message from Darlene.

Darlene: When can you start? I am so happy to have you back.

Jodi: I can start in a week. Gotta wrap things up here first. Thank you so much. One thing, will it be a problem to get July 10-12 off? Scott is in New York and will be coming home. I need to be here.

Darlene: Oh my Jodi, I had no idea, of course, no problem. Send him my thanks and support. Love to you. Can't imagine how tough this has to be for you and your kids.

Jodi: Thank you, Darlene. It is very hard. I appreciate those words more than you know. Another question. How is your PPE supply? Do I need to obtain my own?

Darlene: No, we are doing well. Duke's foundation thankfully has been able to obtain for us. It's not in abundance but it is enough. We are lucky as many hospice agencies or home health agencies are not. Home programs are the 'low man' on the totem pole when it comes to PPE, first priority is the hospitals. Tough all around.

Jodi: That is great. You are so right though in the lucky part. Where I am currently, three masks are to be used for a week with no guarantee of replacement. Scott is telling me where he is at, it is getting slightly better. Still re-using N95s for a week though and keeping your personal allotment in a brown paper bag between shifts. I still can't believe all of this is happening.

I will tell Scott tonight. I know he won't like it but I also know he will understand. Telling the kids will be harder. Is it fair to ask them, or expect them, to be okay with both of us volunteering for positions that puts us at a high risk of contracting the virus? Yeah, not even close to being fair. I will do my best to ease the blow. The big difference is that I will come home on weekends. I am also not in a hospital ass-deep in COVID for thirteen hours straight like Scott. I will have minimal time with people and for the most part, I will be able to distance myself, have enough PPE to keep myself safe, and will be fit tested at Duke for proper N95 fitting.

I will need to watch some YouTube videos on don/doffing PPE. I have never been shown that. Isn't that something? Ten years as a nurse and never been shown how to properly put on and take off PPE. I mean I know how to do it, but to do it to ensure actual protection and not contamination, yeah, no idea. The only time an N95 mask has ever been on my face was in a nursing school demonstration. I haven't been properly fitted to know my size. I don't even know exactly what that entails or how it is done. Just another example of how out of norm this entire situation is. Perhaps once Scott gets settled with my news he can tell me. He has always been my resource for all of this stuff.

But now my own anxiety is creeping in. Those butterflies start their own dance in my belly. Some are excited, many are nervous, and most are anxious. The dance party happening can't be ignored. Can I really do this? Can I really travel to a location, jump into the situation, and be part of a relief crew by myself? Scott has always been by my side since I started travel nursing. Our plan, once the kids were grown, was simple: hit the road together as travel nurses. And for a while, we did just that—living out of suitcases, chasing assignments, sharing the chaos and the purpose.

But about two months ago, we finally started to slow down. We were settling into Myrtle Beach, making it ours. Our place. A home. And just as we began to unpack more than our bags—our hopes, our routines, our future—COVID hit. Hard. Everything shifted. The road we thought we'd left behind came roaring back, only this time, it wasn't an adventure. It was a mission. A reckoning. When we first started traveling together, a little over a year ago, I was unsure I could ever be a travel nurse. Watching him do this for the past thirteen years set the bar high. He never doubted me. Not once. He believed in me and my abilities as a nurse. Fully. Without question. My confidence grew because of his confidence in me and because he was with me. I could text him at any point and ask any question. When I got home, I would debrief every detail and ask more questions. He pushed me to be not just a great travel nurse but a better nurse overall—a better version of myself. He was my mentor. Now, he is in New York and I will be in North Carolina. Both of us alone. But I am determined. I *will* do this. I *can* do this on my own. I will honor him, he taught me well.

...

"Are you fucking kidding me!" he screams as I pick up his call.

"Honey, what are you talking about?"

"I can't even look at Facebook anymore. I was just looking at a feed called, "You Signed Up for This." People just don't get it. They have no idea what is going on. And let me tell you what is being reported is not what I am seeing! It is not old people, with comorbidities of diabetes, being overweight, and whatever else they are saying. My patients, my unit, are young, younger than me, and some as young as our kids. We are renting, yes I said renting, x-ray equipment because there isn't enough and even those rentals aren't enough. And they are not good quality because they are portable. I am putting more people in body bags in one night, hell, the first fucking four hours of a shift than I have in years in ICU. I am putting more people in bags than I have in my entire career as ICU!"

"Honey, please just get off Facebook. You're right, people don't get it, you didn't get it, none of us could get it. And honestly people are stupid and infuriating. You don't deserve this or deserve to even look at it. Are you journaling?" I ask, attempting to change the subject, attempting to calm him before I drop the bomb.

"Yes, I am trying. I am not too consistent, but I am trying. I still can't believe Josh died from all this. He was such a good guy. A wonderful soul."

Silence takes over. He worked with Josh in 2013 during a travel contract at Myrtle Beach, before we called Myrtle

Beach home. Josh was in nursing school at the time, working nights as an ICU tech [nurses aide]. He and Scott became fast friends. Josh was emphatic that we not pass up Bojangles when we moved to Myrtle. His words "KFC has nothin' on Bojangles." He was the kindest man. Josh was exposed to COVID doing what he loved, nursing, and died mid-April 2020.

"I know please be safe. Promise you are taking every precaution there is available," pleading with him.

"I am. I promise. Before I come home, I am getting the blood draw for antibodies. They say it's the most accurate and right now the only thing that is. It will only show if I've had it, not like a positive or negative for COVID," he reports.

"So how do they know now who is COVID positive?" I ask, confused.

"Now it's just by symptoms. Which is the mind-blowing part. And the symptom severity differs for everyone. Some think it's a cold or the flu and wait, thinking it will get better like it has in the past. Some, it takes only a few minutes, some it takes a few hours before shortness of breath starts, by this time it is out of control," he explains.

"Last night I was assigned my one guy that I admitted a few weeks ago. He's been here since March 31st, so it's been almost a month. He had been sick for seven days before coming in. My other patient I was assigned to was able to be weaned from the vent. My first guy is now paralyzed. We medically induce this with medications to keep him from working against the vent. His lungs are so noncompliant. We are seeing this with all of our patients. The guy in Room 45 died, he went into sudden cardiac arrest from hydroxychloroquine they believe. What people don't realize or are not being told is the cardiac effects this has on people. You know me, I have worked in critical care for almost twenty years. This is different. These people aren't dying because they didn't take care of themselves, hell, some that haven't taken care of themselves make it while ones that have are dying. There is no rhyme or reason. No one is immune to this. No one," he says in angry disbelief.

"That is so sad. I don't even know if people know who to believe anymore. There is so much crazy shit coming out of the White House, the news stations, and then add in Facebook gospel land, no one trusts anyone. All the information is contradicting and is confusing. I think most are just scared and don't know what to do and grasp at every word that feels like an answer or justification of their own wishful thinking. Then there are the ones that fall down the rabbit hole of thinking it's all a hoax. Just sad on so many levels. Saddest for you and all the nurses and doctors trying so hard to figure it out," I tell him.

"Yeah I guess. I just wish people would listen. How was your day today?" he asks.

My stomach flips, and my heart picks up its pace. I know that there is no easy or right way to tell him that I'm going back to travel nursing. I just have to say it.

"So I made a decision today," I say trying to sound confident but it comes out more in a question.

"Oh yeah, what's that?" he asks through a chuckle

I take a deep breath and dive in. "I put my notice in," I say, breath catching. "I'm going back to travel at Duke. I already talked with Darlene—she's excited to have me back. They sent the contract. I signed it today. I start April 27th." It all comes out in one exhale.

Silence.

In his mentor's voice he asks, "Are you sure?"

"Yes," I say with a fierce clarity. "I can't sit there in an office and do nothing. My hospice skill set isn't yours—not the ICU adrenaline, not the codes or vents. But mine is needed now too." I pause, letting the truth settle. "More people aren't sick enough to warrant a hospital stay. Or they decide to stay home. Or decide to come home—just to be with family. To not die alone. I'm needed now. I have to try and help." I tell him with the same steadiness that he used when he told me of his decision.

He doesn't speak right away. He exhales slowly. "You know what this means," he says quietly. Not as a warning. Not as a husband, but a fellow responder. The shift is subtle—he is no longer scanning for weakness, but for readiness.

"I do," I say. "Long days. PPE. Families who don't know how to say goodbye. And the weight of it all when I come home."

"I just got used to you being safe," he admits. Then, softer: "I liked knowing where you were."

"I know," I whisper. "But I can't stay behind the glass while people are dying in living rooms. I need to be where I can hold a hand. Maybe I can make it less lonely."

"You have to be safe. Mask all the time. Wash your hands. Gown up when you're told."I'm ordering us some respirator-type masks." he says, pragmatically. "A lot of nurses here have them—they're better than the disposable N95s."

"Disposable?" I scoff. "Oh, you mean the ones that *used* to be disposable and now magically aren't?" The sarcasm slips out before I can stop it.

"Listen to me!" he snaps, voice sharp with worry. "Yes, they come with replaceable filters. But they're more comfortable." He takes a breath so deep I hear it through the phone. "Baby, I knew it wouldn't be long." He pauses, breath catching. "I don't like it. I don't know what I'd do if something happened to you. But I understand. I love you." His voice softens, and I feel it in my chest.

"Thank you," I whisper. "I *will* be safe. Can you explain how they do the fit tests? How do I put on PPE? How do I take it off right?" The questions tumble out like bullets, fast and frantic.

"Hold on, hold on..." he tries to answer. "We'll go over all of it." Then, quieter: "Have you told the kids?"

I shake my head, as if he can see me. "You're the first. I will tonight."

"Okay," his sigh is heavy and exhausted. "Well I'm here at the hospital and about to walk in. I love you. I'll talk to you in the morning." He says with another sigh.

We're both carrying the emotional weight of the conversation and my decision. The only time we can talk by phone is during his nightly walk into work—far from ideal, but better than texting something that deserves to be spoken aloud. So I told him, knowing full well he'd be stepping into the chaos of another shift with this heavy truth now lodged in his chest. And now he's gone, swallowed by the hospital's demands, while I'm left here alone, sitting in the silence, and everything that came with saying it out loud.

I made the mistake of going back and reading the feed on Facebook that had him so angry. "You Signed Up for This." A place where opinions masquerade as truth and empathy gets drowned out by volume. There it was—someone we know. Not a stranger. Not a troll. Someone behind the keyboard, typing with certainty about a situation they've only seen through someone else's lens.

It breaks my heart for Scott. To see friends—family, even—so quick to judge, so far removed from the reality he's living. They speak as if they know. As if headlines and hearsay are enough.

Just ask us, I grumble to myself. *If you want the truth, ask.* But do they really want it? Because the truth isn't clean. It's not convenient. It's not wrapped in a meme or a soundbite. No rainbows and butterflies. The truth is blood and sweat and PPE that digs into your skin. It's holding a hand that's going cold. It's questioning your own worth and whether or not you're doing enough, making any difference at all. It's walking into a room knowing you will not walk out the same.

You can't handle the truth! Jack Nicholson's voice echoes in my head. *A Few Good Men.* One of my all-time favorite movies. And that line—*that* line—is the epitome of how I feel. Because if you could handle the truth, you'd stop typing and start listening.

I don't have the energy for a Facebook fight tonight, or, at all anymore. There are much bigger things to contend with. Telling the kids about what I've decided to do.

CHAPTER 10

Reopening

Today is Madison's twentieth birthday. When I get home she is getting ready to go to her friend's house for her pandemic-style party. Even in a pandemic she harnesses the Me Day excitement. Her energy feels tangible and fills our home with joy. It engulfs me walking through the door. She has no idea how much I need it. She vibrates on such a high level, I can't deny that she single handedly protects this momma's spirit and psyche.

Madison's voice rang out before I even stepped into her room—bright, joyful, unmistakably her. "Momma!" she called, dancing through a sea of clothing choices, prepping for her party. I matched her energy with a "Happy Me Day!" and watched her move with that magnetic spirit she's always carried. She's the kind of soul who asks about your day not out of habit, but out of genuine care. She's been that way since she was little, always wanting those around her to feel loved, seen, happy.

As I watched her, I cast a silent wish: *Never lose your sparkle. Never let anyone dim your shine.*

I hug her, but this time with more weight behind it. I needed to talk to her. The shift was immediate—her smile fading, her tone turned cautious. She asked if Scott was okay, her first instinct since the day he left, always to worry about him. He's never far from her heart, even when she hides it too well.

I reassured her that he was fine. That we'd talked on my drive home. He was headed back to work.

She mentioned he'd texted her happy birthday and seemed surprised, almost guilty for expecting it. I reminded her that of course he would. "You kids are his driving force." Their messages, their voices—they're what keep him going. He tells me that all the time.

Her spirit lifted talking about him coming home in a few months. Then she asked what I needed to tell her.

That's when I hesitated. I'd already made the decision, but now I questioned if I should have talked to her first. I told her I was going back to travel nursing. Duke University had a need, and I could start in a week.

She sat quietly, the sparkle in her eyes dimming. "Are you sure?" she asked.

I was. And she didn't fight it. She told me she was proud of me, even as she held back tears. She said she'd be fine, but I had to be safe—and we had to talk every day.

I promised her I would. I explained how this would be different from Scott's ICU work. I'd be in homes, not hospitals. I'd know what I was walking into. I'd take every precaution. Masks were required. I'd stay in a hotel during the week and come home every weekend.

We hugged, wiped tears, and I nudged her toward her party. Her light returned, just a flicker, but enough. As she grabbed her bag and turned to leave, she asked if I'd be okay.

"I will," I said. "Go have the best time. Be safe. I love you. Happy Me Day!"

I watch her leave and wonder about what the world is going to look like from now on. *Will we ever have "normal" times again? Will we always be wearing a mask? Have birthday parties consisting of only three to four people?* I turn the TV on, the ticker at the bottom continues to scroll. The numbers continue adding more digits, confirmed cases now in the hundreds of thousands. Tens of thousands of deaths. Tens of thousands of people are now no longer with their families because of this. Months into the pandemic and still doesn't feel real. I still cannot comprehend the horrific vastness of it.

The State of New York with 159,937 confirmed cases, it has now surpassed Spain, Italy, and China. NBC reports from CDC data release.

Telling the rest of the kids wasn't as hard as it was when we told them about Scott's decision. They understand the difference in our specialties—Scott is in the ICU, deep in the epicenter of the crisis in New York, surrounded by critical cases and constant exposure. My work is in hospice, and while I'll be bedside again, it's a different kind of bedside. Honestly, it's a little safer.

I'll be in the community, not in a hospital overwhelmed by COVID. There's still uncertainty—who's positive, who's a carrier—but that's no different than how we live now. Going to Walmart or pumping gas carries the same unknowns. The difference is, I'll know my patients' COVID status. Testing is now diagnostic, meaning any suspicion of COVID we now have available home test kits that can provide results within minutes. And most of my visits can be done with social distancing in mind. I won't have the exhaustion of breathing through a mask for thirteen straight hours like Scott does. Between patients, I'll be in my car—I can take the mask off, breathe, reset. And I'll be able to come home each weekend. This made it easier for the kids to accept. It's not without risk, but it's not the same storm Scott battles daily.

The week went quick between making the decision and getting ready to leave. Training modules completed. Hotel reservation made. Packing only for a week. Done. Done. And done.

Arriving to Durham, North Carolina, where Duke is located, was odder, and a bit sadder, than I anticipated. Scott is not with me. The last time I was here, we were here together. Now, I am arriving alone. I drove by our old neighborhood where we stayed during my first contract. I see where we walked Gruxton before and after work. I passed by the restaurant where we ate on the rooftop and talked for hours. Sheetz runs for smoothies, pickled eggs, and smorgasbord for late night driveway talks. Everywhere I look I see him. This whole place is one big Scott memory reel. The loneliness of my heart is heavy. I was starting to get somewhat familiar with him being away from home. It's been close to four weeks of trying to adapt to his lack of presence at home. But now I'm somewhere else, somewhere we built memories, and it feels like him leaving all over again.

Arriving at the hotel was a little eye opening. My requirements for the hotel were simple. I wanted something that was cheap, within good proximity of my patient territory, and it had to be conducive to my coping mechanism, 'smoker friendly'. My expectations were also simple. Clean. A bed, and a small fridge and coffee pot. Outside of that I didn't need any other bells and whistles. Checked in via a barred protected glass, with a metal drawer manually slid out to me to exchange credit card, license, receipt, and key to room. No room in the metal drawer or through the glass for niceties despite my best effort at a smile, hoping I didn't look as intimidated as I was feeling.

The entire world is on alert. The pleasantries shared between strangers—those brief moments that add just a little happiness to our days—are gone. We have physical barriers preventing all of it. Plexi glass, six feet of distance between everyone, masks hiding half our face. Our humanness is being tested and I wonder if it will ever return.

I was thankful that my room was at the very end and I could park right outside my door. I had no way of trying to blend in with the residents of the hotel. My Jeep with 'Moon Momma' plastered on the side made me stick out. It was obvious I wasn't in the most affluent area of Durham. Once I got inside, my routine checks began. Fridge works. The bed, however, causes a slight pause, the outer cover, full of burn holes, dingey, and smelling of who knows what. The entire room carried the fragrance of month-old Marlboros. It was enough to cause me to pause and recognize that this wasn't going to be the most comfortable of stays. But, I don't have the energy to care. I brought my own quilt and pillows and would make a quick trip to get some candles to use along with my packed diffuser. Bathroom was next, it was surprisingly cleaner than I had expected. All-in-all, I was good. Still not the best feeling in my gut about the place, but I would make it work for the week.

Scott always took care of finding our accommodations. I never ever worried whether or not somewhere was safe when I was with him. He always made sure that it was. I'll just keep repeating to myself that it is fine, it's just for a week, I'll be away working most of the time. I laugh thinking that there is no way that I could be accused of being "boujie" staying in a place like this. Thankful for the conversations and affirmations with myself; it helps with the density of loneliness that seems to be a constant companion these days. Being isolated and away from everyone actually feels okay. I don't have to pretend or be on guard. I can just be with myself, in all my unsettled, anxious, sad, and lonely energy.

My wrist dings, my watch alerting me to an incoming call from Scott.

"Hey, Baby," he says, "Whatcha doing?" The words are upbeat but his tone is exhausted. Every time I hear his voice I can feel his weariness and the heaviness of his soul despite his efforts to hide it from me, and perhaps himself.

I respond in the most confident, upbeat way that I can letting him know that I'm checked into the hotel and getting settled in. My sole mission is to stay positive, to not add any further worry or stress for him. This is my attempt to help keep his spirits as high as possible. We're both trying to protect each other from what we're feeling and experiencing. We're both intentionally hiding parts of our lives to keep a level of normalcy in our conversations and create a safe space to just *be* for a moment.

He starts the call with a bit of humour. "Last night I had a doctor try to report off to me, thinking I was the oncoming doctor." He chuckles. "I let it go for a bit, before I told him that I was a nurse."

"Well I can certainly understand his confusion, you are so beyond, in so many ways, the expectation that many have of what a 'typical nurse' is," I tell him proudly.

"Thank you, Baby, but no, it's not that. It's more like we are all one. None of the initials matter now, we are all just trying to save lives." He sighs, dropping into seriousness now. "None of it matters, nothing is working. We gather around every night, all of us, docs, nurses, respiratory, PAs, all of us, scratching our heads. Throwing out options, like a Jeopardy game. "Give me ventilation setting for 200, Alex." We have tried it all, every single thing they are telling us that has had *some* hopeful outcome. Vitamin C, Vitamin D, Zinc. Hydroxychloroquine, antibody infusions. We aren't picky, if there has been some measure of success, we're trying it. We have gone back and forth, over and over. It feels like we are relearning our medical background all over and on the fly. The advancement of your degree doesn't matter. It's worthless now, we are all in a foreign battle, side by side, and just as clueless as the person standing next to us. This is what no one sees, no one understands. And honestly no one believes." He sounds utterly disgusted and dejected.

"We have a core group, they are family now," he continues. "We are good together. You know Dr. Kochan, then the nurses Brett from Oklahoma, Kim, from Ohio, and D'Navi, we call her Shaq, we just found out that she is pregnant. Saint

Louis, the nurse from Texas, she is usually my desk buddy. Her and Shaq are Krucial nurses. Alvin is like the class clown of the unit. He is usually always smiling and tries his best to keep us all smiling and laughing at some point. He has started making these funny masks. He takes the surgical masks that we have to wear over our N95s and puts mouths on them, like teeth and shit. He says that because it's what the patient sees he figured he could make that a little more fun for them and us. That tells you what kinda guy he is."

"He laughs about my meals, they all do, but now he is asking me all kinds of questions about keto and the benefits. I have started working with him on it. He calls me the "keto guru". Oriana, is a NP, she is from Colorado. It's weird, I mean I have made friends at every assignment, but this group is different. I feel deeply bonded to them. We connected instantly. There wasn't hesitation, but really there was no time either. If there is any comfort or confidence to be had, this group is it." His gratitude is palpable.

"Baby, I am glad that you have them. Of course, the connection is different, you guys are in the fight together, none of us know what that is like. It will be a bond that ties you all together long after this. Hey, ask Alvin if he can, I would love him to send me two funny masks. I have a patient now that I would love to give it to. I talk about you and where you are all the time with her. She always tells me, "Tell him to stay safe and thank you," I say.

"Okay, Baby, I will ask him." His mood shifts. "I can't believe they're even talking about reopening?!" Anger now. "What the fuck is wrong with people? We're still in a PPE shortage—including fucking body bags. So hey, let's open it up?! What the fuck!" He finishes sarcastically, then falls into silence again.

Reopening. The word itself feels reckless. It means lifting restrictions, letting people flood back into stores, into restaurants—while the virus still lingers, still spreads. For Scott, standing in the ICU, reopening isn't a policy debate. It's a threat. It's more patients. More ventilators. More lives slipping through his gloved hands.

For me, his wife, reopening means he won't come home—not until the cases stop. Not until the curve bends. Not until the world decides that lives matter more than convenience.

"I know," trying not to vocally match his anger. "We just have to have faith that people will continue to do the right thing."

"Faith..." he mutters. "Faith? Yeah, that is long gone.

Faith in people? Have you looked at Facebook recently? He says acrimoniously. "Complaining about wearing a mask, talking about 'it's against my rights'. Saying they can't breathe. It's just like the flu or it's a hoax. Let me tell them about wearing a mask suctioned to your face for thirteen hours a day and breathing... I haven't taken a full breath, with or without a damn mask, for weeks now. Like the flu, a hoax? Come to Elmhurst and then tell me just how much like the flu it is and that it's a hoax! Let me show you how many body bags I zip up in one shift. Come volunteer to hold a real person's hand. Come try and reassure them as they gasp for every breath, knowing that it is only a matter of time before they will end up on a ventilator. We know the odds of coming off that ventilator, *yeah, assholes, it's low*. We don't leave them. Here is your fucking hoax!" The despair and fury in his voice hits my heart like a gunshot.

Telling him that I'm sorry and that I love him is all I can muster after that. What else can I say? Nothing that will help. Even "I'm proud of you" feels hollow now. It used to mean something—admiration, respect, love. But now? It feels like a betrayal. Like I'm standing on the sidelines, clapping, while he drowns.

Yes, I'm proud. Fiercely. But pride feels shallow against

the brutality of what he's enduring. I'm angry—at the world, at the recklessness, at every person who shrugs this off like it's over. They don't see him. They don't see the body bags, the sweat-soaked masks, the haunted eyes. They don't see what it costs to a human spirit, his spirit, to will someone to keep breathing.

So no, I'm not just proud. I'm wrecked. I want to scream at every reopened door, every crowded bar, every careless smile I see because they're not wearing a mask. I want to face-punch every mouth that dares to say, *"It's just like the flu." "It's not real." "Masking violates my rights."*

Because while they move on, he stays behind—fighting for strangers who may never even know his name. Holding the hands of those who once spewed hatred and ignorance across a keyboard. Calming the fears of patients who whisper, "I wish I had listened. I was one of them." And that's what breaks me. Not just the injustice, but the grace he offers in the face of it. He keeps showing up.

I try so hard to imagine what it's like, to find some thread of understanding. I want to relate to him, to reach him, to heal him. But try as I might, I know I never will. Only those Elmhurst COVID warriors carry this cross. Only they know the weight.

And they will bear it—for the rest of their lives.

CHAPTER 11

Spies Among Us

END OF APRIL GOING INTO MAY 2020

Life is a compilation of stories—ours, theirs, the ones we tell ourselves to sleep at night, and the ones we're forced to swallow whole. These stories shape our truths. They become our beliefs. Because reality isn't a fixed point—it's a lens, a very personal lens colored by experience, fear, hope, or agenda. Perception is also very personal which makes it fragile. When circumstances shift—when grief, chaos, or doubt creep in—it's easy to see the world differently. We're human. We crave answers. We reach for *why* like it's a lifeline. But sometimes, the search for truth becomes a weapon. Sometimes, the story someone brings with them isn't meant to heal—it's meant to fracture.

I just wish someone, healthcare workers, leaders, anyone with influence, would just stand up and say it plainly: We do not know. *We do not know!!* Medical clinicians of every type, every specialty, every discipline have always been looked to for sound advice, to offer guidance to help people make the best decisions for their health. But now? We can't offer that. We're just as uncertain. Just as afraid. We don't know what exactly we're dealing with or why, and that uncertainty is paralyzing. Everyone is reeling from the reality in front of us.

There is another press conference with the President today. I haven't missed one. In April he said, "And then I see the disinfectant, where it knocks it out in a minute... Is there a way we can do something like that, by injection inside or almost, a cleaning?"

It is so hard to listen to these now. I cannot believe that we have politicized a health pandemic, but that is exactly what is happening. Am I hearing the President of the United States instructing people to inject themselves with bleach and Lysol. To insert UV light into the body. *The next shortage will undoubtedly be light sabers.* I shouldn't be, but I sit here in disbelief. This is the President for God's sake saying this all while medical leaders, standing shoulder to shoulder with him, say nothing. I truly cannot believe I am hearing this, living this. No accountability, no empathy to the hundreds of thousands of lives being lost, alone. No "thank you" to the thousands of healthcare workers. No responsible or evidence-based guidance whatsoever. It's delusional, almost word salad. It's confusing to the masses.

"They have no idea what is going on," Scott tells me over and over again. Pleading to me, but really crying out for someone, anyone, to listen.

Everywhere you look—online, in-person, on social media, everyone is looking to blame someone, something. It has been six weeks since the U.S. has spiked with infections and we are all still trying to wrap our brains around the numbers that still haven't plateaued. All of us are an unsettled mix of feelings: vulnerable, scared, and in denial, combined with holding out hope that answers could be right around the corner. The Internet is both a soothing mechanism and a catalyst for making things worse. It is so easy to "quickly" go online to get an update or any new information and just as quickly find yourself down a rabbit hole spending hours getting yourself so emotionally worked up that your already overextended nervous system feels even more battered. I am not exempt from the rabbit holes. I fall down regularly.

Just go to bed, my brain chatter interjects tonight, like every night. *Stop looking.* But like a train wreck, as the saying goes, I can't look away. When I finally fall asleep I wake a short time later to the sound of my phone ringing and vibrating right off the table. With Scott away I never turn off my notifications so even my rest isn't restful. One ear is always listening. Tonight, it is BFF and she is going off the hook. She texted me a YouTube link to a video called "The Undercover Nurse." She follows this up with three words. "Spyglasses. Watch this!"

Hesitantly I click the link. The video starts playing. It is an interview being conducted with a nurse who is working at Elmhurst. She is talking about working there and how care is not being performed correctly, patients being put on ventilators that don't need them and, I am summarizing, that the nurses are "killing these patients." WHAT!!!! She is showing patient charts, not redacted, talking with fellow colleagues, one being BFF, about patients and how she got this video from the "inside." She proceeds to tell that she wore spyglasses to gather all this information. Glasses that to the naked eye appeared to be normal eyeglasses, except hers had a hidden camera installed. BFF was mortified, angry, hurt, scared. BFF's texts come flying in one right after the other.

BFF: I didn't know she was taping me.

She didn't know how to suction a vent, she questioned everyone including the docs about everything.

None of us knew.

What am I supposed to do?

The messages are coming through faster than I can read them. Now Scott starts texting.

Scott: Got a message from the hospital CEO and nurse managers telling us to not look like a nurse when coming to and from work. We are to wear street clothes from now on. We were told we are getting death threats and that they know when we arrive and leave for work. That's what I woke up to today.

Now I feel like I'm playing Whac-A-Mole between the two of them, trying to keep up. I can't even respond fast enough. I hear the fear from BFF and the anger and outrage from Scott. Each phone vibration from the incoming texts is a jolt running through my fingers directly to my heart.

Scott: Walking to work now, no more cheers, no more clashing of the pans, no more thank you. Now, it's angry comments, disbelievers, fighting amongst each other. The trust we work so hard to gain, destroyed in one day.

I feel his defeat reading his words.

Scott: We are doing everything and nothing is working.

I feel him cracking as his words continue.

Scott: Every fucking night all of us, the docs, nurses, NPs, respiratory therapists, we still gather every night and go over what we tried, brainstorming what else we can try, all of us are doing everything we know. It's like a war room many times throughout a shift. It always ends in frustration from all of us. Adrenaline never goes away or down. Some literally look like they are crashing, none of us are sleeping on days off. That's laughable to even say, 'days off.'

I can't see him, but I envision him laughing in an evil tone. My phone rings, I almost drop it, when I answer he continues.

"There are no days off, we are consumed, trying to figure it out, what will work, what if *this* or what if *that*, cause we all know that everything we have trained for, is not working! All of us come in with dark circles and heavy bags holding up our eyeballs, that are glazed over with exhaustion. Our noses are shiny as we add another coat of Vasoline, skin prep, or whatever else we think might lessen the sting of our nose bridges. Hell, we would be happy with an hour of any kind of relief. Our cheeks dry, chapped, and red, some with open sores from the fucking vice grip of the mask straps. We walk into that war room many times every night trying everything we can think, everything within our power to help everyone, all while we sit and wonder if we have it, too. At this point, we are so exhausted and consumed from trying to save everyone, we would miss our own early signs. I look around, some are crying, and some don't even know they are because we've become accustomed to wiping the silent tears that fall each day. I have seen some completely lose it, the ugly cry that is uncontrollable. We are so vulnerable like this. Relying on each other to try to get through this and now we have to wonder if we can even trust each other."

This is another one of those moments when there isn't anything to say aside from offering him my unwavering support. The tears are silently falling down my face just like those in the war room. And just like them, mine are laced with disgust that someone would betray the selflessness, the courage, and the care that all these frontline workers are giving. In this moment, the tears are hot, burning as they leave my eyes and trek down my cheeks. Fury escaping me along with my tears. This is personal. My husband is one of them—one of the few who run toward the fire while others flee. A frontline worker who walks into chaos night after night, not for glory, not for recognition, but because saving lives is stitched into the fabric of who he is. He suits up knowing the risks, knowing the toll, knowing that each shift might ask more of him than the last. He's held hands through final breaths, whispered comfort through masks, and carried the weight of families who couldn't be there. He is not just fighting a virus—he's fighting despair, injustice, and the crushing reality that even heroes break. And still, he goes back. Because the world needs him. Because he refuses to let it fall apart without a fight. He is not alone, the core crew as he refers to them, Dr. Kochan, Alvin, Saint. Louise, Shaq, Bret, Nicole, Kim, Latasha, and BFF have sacrificed so much and so much more yet to be realized by any of them.

"I worry about Shelia [BFF]," he tells me. "I am really proud of her though. I was unsure how and if she would be able to handle it. Now with this spyglasses bullshit, I am worried about her. I don't blame her for being irate, I would be too. I am glad I didn't have any interaction with that woman. What that person has caused for a few bucks and her one minute of fame is disgusting. What she fails to show is the truth. She doesn't show how for thirteen hours we are chickens with our heads cut off. She doesn't show that we're coding people who are in their twenties, thirties, forties, fifties... routinely, every shift, multiple times in a shift. You know these are not the ages of people who get coded. There are refrigerated tractor trailers to hold the bodies because the morgue can't hold enough. She doesn't talk about all of that, does she? We get assignments, but that means nothing, we are all working all the patients in the exact same way because there isn't time to do anything else. Propofol, Levophed, and Fentanyl on top of carts, because there isn't time for the pharmacy to fill our medication machines, because we are emptying them faster than they can stock. The ongoing chaos of coding a patient when the crash cart is already in use for another one. This is what is happening. This is what no one wants to hear. And the reality of all of this sure as hell isn't gonna make for a good headline or make someone famous or wealthy. I am not enough, we are not enough." Silence holds the space of that admission as he arrives back at the hospital for another grueling shift.

What more can happen? my heart voice asks. *I am not enough, we are not enough* repeats in my head. Has this country completely lost their minds? Poor BFF. Her jolliness. Her excited nature about everything. Her pride in her skill set. Her silly nicknames for everything. She loves with her whole soul. Her light is already flickering by COVID, but now this woman with the spyglasses is extinguishing it all for a few clicks on the Internet. The *real* heroes, the *real* warriors, now have to battle outside of the hospital too. And for what? Her selfishness. Her carelessness. As if everyone needed this on top of everything else.

CHAPTER 12

"You Are My Friend"

END OF MAY THROUGH JUNE 2020

Our reality is dim. They are working on getting more tests so everyone can be tested. But for now, these too are limited and rationed out. Priority is given to our older population, nursing homes, people at high risk for infection, cancer, lung issues, and more. Here is the kicker: High risk does not include healthcare workers so we all still just sit and wonder when we'll be next. It is always a *when, never* an *if.*

My call from Scott that day has me cautiously smiling. His "Hey, Baby" when I answer the phone is a bit more upbeat than it's been in weeks. He tells me that he wants to tell me about his night. Upbeat and talking about a shift are not normally associated, so I'm hesitant with my response.

"Okay..."

"Remember my guy, he was sixty-one from El Salvador? He has been in the hospital since the end of March."

It is now the beginning of May, so this patient has been in the hospital for many weeks. He proceeds to remind me of how sick he was, the meds they were trying with him, and even the trial research drug he was on. I recall it all because this one patient has been a patient of Scott's since he first got to Elmhurst nearly two months ago.

"He had been progressively getting worse. His oxygen levels continued to decrease despite multiple modalities of delivery resulting in intubation since he couldn't breathe on his own. Most of the patients we have been seeing who get to this point, have a high rate of mortality. He required proning when he could tolerate it. He had to be medically sedated and paralyzed to allow the vent work. He is now at the point we are trying to wake him and hopefully extubate and take him off the ventilator. The doctors have been weaning him with big jumps, like going from 180 to dead stop."

I interrupt, confused. "Babe, you have to dumb this down, I am not an ICU nurse and have no idea what this means."

"Okay," and begins an explanation in a grade school teacher tone. "Proning means turning them onto their stomachs to help improve oxygen levels. We have a full team dedicated for just this, meaning the entire shift, this is all they do. The team consists of eight people, all Air force deployments, usually a doctor and/or anesthesiologist with the rest made up of respiratory therapists. They execute this with such precision, almost surgical, as you could imagine. The patients are unresponsive, on many medications through IVs, on a ventilator, so lots of tubes, lines. So, in a very fragile, clinical state. It has to be performed with synchrony. Honestly, it looked almost ceremonial. The entire process would take them ten to fifteen minutes. Well, I can't explain it more than that, but I'm sure you understand now," he continued my lesson.

"Weaning from the ventilator is just as it sounds, but in these circumstances it requires a slow steady decrease of both the paralytic medications and the ventilator settings that have been keeping them alive. We decrease the meds and the vent settings and watch to see how their heart is handling the changes and if their lungs are able to breathe without machines and/or medications. If they can't breathe easily we will see heart rates increase, respirations increase, oxygen levels decrease and overall, the patient will be scared and restless because they feel like they can't breathe. You can only imagine how scary this would be, when their last memory is breathing normally."

Lesson complete. For a moment there it was like when I would come to him in the evenings of my travel nurse assignments and debrief with him and ask him to clarify or explain something to me. And, as always, I am so impressed with how he explains everything so that it is understood. He really is such a wonderful nurse. I am in awe of him.

"So back to last night," he shifts his tone, sounding almost excited. "I just told them I was going to handle the weaning. Long story short, the settings were off and when we tried to wake him he was clearly uncomfortable. I asked the resident to switch the modes and he responded: 'We don't do things like this overnight.' I being me, said 'WTF does that mean? He is awake and is uncomfortable and I am not knocking him back out with sedation.' The resident says he would go look at the chart and see what the day doctors have been doing. I went back into the patient room and held his hand trying to talk him through it. Trying to calm him. I explained what was happening, so that he understood. Ten minutes passed. I went and found Dr. Kochan. I explained what was happening, what had been working, and told him what I wanted to do to make the patient more comfortable without sedating him again. Dr. Kochan said it sounded like a great idea, for me to make the setting switch and he would go put the orders in for it. I ran back to the room, made the switch. I sat there watching. His heart rate came down from 120 to 90, his blood pressure came down, and his respiratory rate came down but not quite enough so I gave him a bit more pressure support until he looked comfortable. I wrote down the settings and gave them to the resident telling him that I just put these vent orders in from Dr. Kochan. He looked at me like I just pissed in his Cheerios."

He laughs and continues. "When I left this morning my patient was awake. He was weak but awake and breathing. I hope we can get him extubated." I can hear the slight sense of hope in his voice. "I need a success story, Baby," he adds in an exhausted exhale.

We get off the phone so he can get some sleep. I find myself in a silent conversation encouraging this patient to breathe, affirming that he's got this and that I would help him from afar. *"Breathe,"* I whisper. *"You've got this. I will help you."* I visualize connecting my breaths to his, helping him steady his breathing until he can breathe on his own again. This one man, fighting for his own survival, doesn't realize he's also fighting for something greater—for the spirit of every nurse who's held a hand, adjusted a mask, whispered encouragement through exhaustion. In his struggle to live, he becomes a quiet symbol of resilience, reminding them why they keep showing up. He's proof that even in the darkest moments, hope can still flicker. His fight says, without words to those who refuse to give up on him, "You ARE enough.".

I am so glad I am on my way home after the week away. Two nights of sleeping in my own bed sounds great. Madison calls me as I am almost home. She sounds tired. She works outside and it has been so hot recently. Wearing the mask all day in the heat makes it extra tiring.

I still can't believe that Topgolf is open in Myrtle Beach. Well, I can, as most in our town are riding the hoax-theory bus. Most don't wear a mask, only follow social distance rules because they are being forced to by the space between chairs, queues, aisles. When I get home, I find her asleep in her bed. I leave her. She looks so peaceful. Even at twenty I still see my baby girl. I make myself a coffee and go to the porch. The silent night is welcoming. My spirit doesn't feel quite as heavy sitting here under the golden Edison lights. Being away from home during the week is just another level making this whole situation taxing.

"Mom," I hear coming from inside. "I am itching, can you look at this?"

She raises her shirt exposing her side. My breath leaves me in an instant. I check her back and see it's there too. A flaming rash that is covering her entire body. I run and get the thermometer. Shove it in her mouth. 100.1. No! No! No! I ask if they've been checking temperatures at work like is required. They have. She tells me it's been 97, 98, and then 99. Since it is so hot out, and 99 degrees isn't considered a temperature, they had her continue working.

My nursing-mode has fully kicked in now. Question after question comes flying out of my mouth. I ask if she's been eating.

"Not really."

I ask if food had a taste when she did.

"I don't know, I wasn't really paying attention."

She sounds like she's apologizing for the lack of having better answers so I assume my face looks worried. Trying to correct my expression, calmly, I tell her to go take an oatmeal bath in hopes it will soothe the itching.

I hear her start the bath. I run down to my Jeep and get my nursing bag, get out my pulse oximeter and stethoscope to listen to her lungs, and check her heart rate and oxygen levels. My insides already know. All I can think about is how I can't take her to the hospital, that I have to do everything I can to keep her home. I can't let her be there alone without me. My nursing credentials would do nothing in this situation. She would be isolated just like every other patient admitted.

I head back inside, check on her and see that this rash is not getting better. I take her temperature and it's increased slightly, now 100.2. She is visibly tired. I get her into bed and get her some juice, along with her tumbler full of water. I bring in something for her to taste so I can see if she can tell me what it is, blind taste test style. I ask her to taste what I have on this spoon and tell me what it is. She opens her mouth and I put the spoon full of Frank's hot sauce in her mouth. I watch for any reaction. None. She says she can't taste it.

As soon as those words leave her mouth, she realizes. The downfall of having two nurses as parents, she knows exactly what is happening. Her eyes are now full of fear. She doesn't want to go to the hospital. She doesn't want to be away from me. She begs me not to make her go. We are fully aligned in this desire, so I hug her and tell her we will do everything we can to avoid going.

I immediately want Scott. He would be the person to help us with this plan and tell us what to do. But, of course, he's dealing with his own daily crises in the middle of his shift so I temper how to approach this with him. Sending him a general, 'hope your night wasn't awful' text is how I decide to open the conversation. I don't want to immediately sound an alarm.

He responds quickly, thank heavens.

Scott: Not worse, not better, same outcomes. When we got to the hospital my heart dropped. There were so many ambulances, firetrucks, and police cars. They all had their lights on. We didn't know what was happening. When I got to the unit, I was told it was a vigil, paying tribute to an ER nurse that died from COVID.

I feel numb. Deep sympathy washes over me. Of course we all know it is a very real possibility. It is the exact reason we were so upset when Scott volunteered. But the reality of it, and right before his shift...I wonder how long it takes before the illusion of safety begins to crack. Before the layers of training, credentials, and protective gear stop feeling like armor and start feeling like sheer curtains. We walk into these roles believing we're prepared, believing we're shielded by knowledge and protocol. But then reality hits—a patient crashes, a colleague gets sick, a loved one volunteers for the frontlines—and suddenly, that deep sense of security we've clung to feels fragile. COVID doesn't care about titles or experience. It strips away the comfort of control, leaving us exposed in ways we never imagined. COVID is not discriminating.

I battle the urge to not tell him about Madison. I attempt to justify my change in subject, telling myself he would want to know. And the truth is, I really need his expertise right now, so I tell him.

Jodi: Madison has a fever, a rash on her entire torso, it is itchy. I gave her hot sauce, didn't tell her what it was, no reaction to the spoonful. We made an appointment to have a test tomorrow.

I send the text with as little emotion but as much detail as possible, as if reporting off at the end of a shift.

Scott: OH MY GOD!! She has COVID!

His fear is tangible. The text bubbles seem to mimic his panic. Bouncing. Stopping. Disappearing. Bouncing again. My fears are now expanding. I can't contain my own thoughts so I send back: He's getting worked up so I try to remain calm.

Jodi: I know. What do I do? What am I looking for? I have to keep her home, I can't send her to the hospital, they won't let me be with her but I have to know when to go.

Scott: Is she having any breathing issues, any at all?

I give him all the details. Temperature. Oxygen (92) and heart rate (88) numbers. Location of the rash. And then the oatmeal bath for the itch and the Tylenol for pain.

Scott: Keep watching O2, if it goes below 90, Baby, you have to take her. Continue with the Tylenol, cool cloths to her head and armpits to help with fever. Go get Zinc, Vitamin C and Vitamin D.

Jodi: I am scared, Baby. I am so sorry that I have to ask all this, it's the last thing you need. But I don't trust anyone else.

I respond heartbroken and scared all the same.

Scott: Keep me posted, watch her closely, even through the night. Make sure they get a good swab tomorrow. They need to go deep, it will feel like they touched her brain. It has to be both nostrils, too. If her eyes don't water it is not a good test sample. Shit, I have to go. Code Blue.

...

"CODE BLUE" blares across the unit. He jumps and runs. No time or space to process that his own daughter increased the ticker scroll by one today or to hold reverence for a fallen fellow COVID warrior. I realize there are no words and I have no idea what this must feel like for him. It is most likely something that I will never be able to understand.

...

Madison and I made it through the night. Her oxygen levels maintained in the low 90s. Her temperature broke and returned several times overnight. The rash remained. Both of us are feeling nervous as we head to the testing site this morning. I know the result in my gut but I'm doing everything I can to remain optimistic. Madison sits silently in the passenger's seat just staring out the window. I feel her fear. We approach the line of cars, directions plastered across makeshift signs, directing us like a Chick-fil-A drive thru. Nurses garbed up as if they are about to take their first moon walk.

It is so hard to wrap my brain around all of this. I feel my heartbeat speed up, the weight sitting on my chest. All I can do is just reach for her hand and softly tell her, "It's going to be okay." Her eyes beam at me in disbelief.

The nurse approaches her window, motions for her to pull her mask down, and lean her head back. Madison follows directions. Quick. Aggressive. Her head jerks back as the swab plunges deep. Tears streak down her face involuntarily. Her eyes stay wide, stunned more by the violation than the pain. "Results by end of day," they mutter through the layers of plastic and fabric. "Watch the portal. If positive, we'll call." We nod. There's nothing else to do. They motion for us to leave.

But we stay—just for a moment. The silence in the car is heavy, like the air inside a sealed capsule. Neither of us speaks. There's nothing to say. Being swabbed through a window by someone shrouded in protective layers feels less like medicine, more like an alien ritual. It's a warped reality dressed in PPE—a sterile invasion, this sci-fi display.

We drive off, blinking against the light of early morning. Somehow, everything feels different now. Another unfathomable layer of this dystopian scene Ten minutes into the ride home she gets an alert to her phone. POSITIVE.

Scott: Good morning, Baby, did you get her tested?

My watch alerts me of his incoming message. With a heavy heart and unsteady fingers I respond and tell him it is positive. He asks how she's doing.

Jodi: She is scared, I won't be going to work. I have to tell them even though I have no symptoms. I couldn't live with myself if I exposed someone. I would assume I would have to be tested and would have to quarantine for ten days. I think that is the policy there.

Scott: Yeah probably. Tell her I love her, and we will be okay.

I'm gonna call you, I have to tell you about my night.

Text is hard at times to determine if this is a time for my heart to drop or speed up in excitement, so mine does both.

"Hey Honey," I answer. "What happened?" I ask with caution.

"Remember my El Salvadoran guy I was telling you about the other day?" His voice is smiling. I haven't heard this happy tone from him in months. "We were able to get him extubated and off the vent. It's been six weeks and last night I went in to introduce myself. I told him I'd been taking care of him for about three weeks and he looked up at me with a smile on his face and said, 'I know, you are my friend.' This morning I was able to get him out of bed and up into the recliner chair. I had to use the hoyer, the machine that helps with lifting a patient that is unable to stand and transfer on their own, because he is still very weak. But, Baby, he was out of that bed! He has a long road to recovery, probably will need a stop at rehab for several weeks, but he is the first one that I've seen go from where he was to getting better. He is one of the 12% that have made it off the ventilator. Today was the victory I needed, that we all needed." His voice cracks.

Choking back tears for both my husband and his patient. "Ahh, that is the best news," unable to contain the small glimmer of hope I'm feeling.

My tears break free as I remember the silent prayer and visual I offered for this patient. *You did it. Thank you. Thank you!* Overwhelmed with gratitude. This one man—this one patient, single-handedly tied a knot in Scott's last fraying thread of hope. He gave Scott something to hold onto. A reason to believe again.

"Baby, you *are* enough," I hear my own voice echo back to me. Words I've said before. Words I'll keep saying. *Mr. El Salvador,* you *are my friend,* my heart tells him. *Thank you.*

I think of the hashtag, #ElmhurstStrong—once just a rallying cry on social media—now it carries the weight of something sacred. It's not just a slogan. It's a badge of survival. Of grace. Of grit. For both patients and nurses, doctors, all of them. I smile through the tears still falling. "Yep," I whisper. "Mr. El Salvador and Scott—both warriors in this COVID war. #ElmhurstStrong."

CHAPTER 13

Leaving Elmhurst

END OF JUNE 2020, BEGINNING OF JULY 2020

Scott's morning call delivers some interesting news.

Well... I guess they think it's getting better. They sent about forty Krucial nurses home. Last night, we said goodbye to Dr. Kochan." His voice was quiet, but heavy.

I could hear the shift in his tone—reverent, a little raw.

"He wasn't loud, you know? Not ego-driven. Just this calm humbleness we all needed. When we gathered around him, no one spoke. He stood in the center of our circle, and we all just... felt it. The loss. The gratitude. He didn't want speeches or applause—actually looked kind of embarrassed by the little send-off we tried to give him."

Scott paused, then added, "His mask was creased from hours of wear, his eyes glassy—exhaustion, emotion, both. We stood there in silence, in reverence. Every time a patient died, no matter how chaotic things were, he made us stop. Bow our heads. Take a quiet breath. A life, honored. He held just as many hands as we did."

I could feel Scott remembering the first time they met. "I saw him drop his military fatigue backpack, name tape showing, and I thought, 'Here we go... another egotistical military doc.' But he wasn't like that. Not even close."

Then his voice softened even more. "Tonight, I was checking on a patient and noticed something in his hand. It was a Ziplock bag with a pocket-sized Bible inside. I asked around—turns out it was Dr. Kochan. He placed one in the hands of four patients who've been here the whole time he was—eight weeks, still on vents. He wrote something personal in each one. Signed them. He didn't just work here. He was one of us. I'm gonna miss him."

"Is it getting better, really?" I ask, wishful.

"The hospital still is all COVID. I wouldn't say anything is improving virus-wise, we are just getting better in managing it," he tells me.

Disappointed, I just remain silent.

"I worry we are opening up things too soon. I don't believe we have a handle on it to keep it mitigated. And then all the ones that still believe a hoax and that won't wear a mask. Yeah, I think we are headed in a bad direction."

I agree. It does feel too soon to open things back up. I don't even know how to feel sometimes. I am angry at all the misleading and confusing information being provided. I don't trust many people. I am sad because of the self-centeredness of people. I fear we will never be *"normal"* again. I even question that. *Normal.* Was it ever really *normal*?"

"I am scheduled to get my antibodies drawn and will be able to get a test before I leave to come home. These next two weeks can't go fast enough," he says.

I am so excited. I cannot wait to see him. We're all excited. He deserves a break from it all. I know COVID has desecrated his spirit so hopefully being back home with us will help, at least a bit. It will be a homecoming celebration, yes, but my priority will also be to help him heal.

"I will be glad to sleep in my own bed. To see you and the kids and my bully boy [Gruxton]."

I sense detachment in his tone. When your only communication for the past three months has been through phone calls, texts, and FaceTime, you become a master at listening for the nuances in tone. He has become an unknowing master at word manipulation for both of us. I wonder if it's intentional or not. Maybe if he gives voice to his words, he can somehow attempt to believe them. An unconscious survival of sanity, perhaps. It is his tone, his inflections of words, the sighs of exhaustion and defeat between statements, the force of his speech, the cadence and enunciation of his words—all of it tells a truth that isn't reflected in what he's saying.

I miss him. And I realize that I am grieving the person he was before he left. I know that with every exhausted sigh, every burst of anger, every moment of despair, has changed him to his core. *Let me be enough to help heal him,* pleading to myself.

...

The next few weeks Madison and I begin our preparations for his homecoming. Madison recovers, pretty much unscathed. It feels like a miracle. She still can't taste or smell and it's been over a month. I fortunately have had no symptoms, along with a negative test, and am able to return to work after ten days off. Kailee in her very Fancyway informs us she also tested positive: "I think it was like one of those false positive pregnancy tests. I don't have any symptoms. They are saying that many are getting false positives with the tests," she tells me. Part of me finds humor in her rationalization of her supposed false positive while the other part is *momma mad* because she isn't taking the result seriously. Thankful, but not surprised, that only two of our kids have tested positive–Madison and Kailee. Those two have always been the ones to be sick, Madison especially. Poor kid gets everything coming and going and twice as worse as anyone else.

Madison and I have decided to get balloons and create a basket of all his favorite things. We will make an "elmhurststrong" banner to drape along the porch balcony. We want everyone to know the hero that resides here. We plan to get the pups bathed, the hardest chore of all and full of drama—Gruxton hates maintenance of any kind.

It is true that our fur babies feel what is happening in their worlds. For the past few months, Gruxton has shown us just how real this is. He now lays for endless hours outside our bedroom door instead of his normal couch spot. We find him at the door every night around 8 p.m., waiting for Scott. After an hour, he sulks to the porch, head down, his tail nub motionless, releasing the most heartfelt sigh of sadness as he belly-plops down, still watching for him to come home. With every car door closing and car alarm setting, his ears perk up and he looks. I imagine him asking: *"Is it Daddy?"*

only to drop his head back down knowing it's not. Scott misses him so much, *"I hope he remembers me."* I reassure him that will not be an issue.

Some nights when Madison is in bed and it's just Grux and I on the porch, we have full blown conversations. He has witnessed so many tears of mine and I have literally wiped his. He is always part of mine and Scott's conversations. Scott always talks to him on the phone, his ears perk up and forward and his eyes smile in excitement when he hears Scott's voice, and then he runs to the door. It is both adorable and heartbreaking. *"It isn't time yet buddy, it won't be long and Daddy will be home,"* his head drops, and he sulkily walks on my heels back to the porch. Grux is my protector, our walks are rarely leisurely anymore. Neither of us are feeling carefree and he is on-guard way too much in Scott's absence. I send Scott pictures all the time because one of the greatest things our boy can do is light up any situation or mood.

The chime of my watch alerts me to incoming call. It's Scott. Now that coming home is in sight, our conversations have a different tone. He tells me about a package he's expecting. A jacket that he ordered from someone with the EMS. And a package that is arriving for me. The masks that Alvin made for us. Only seven more days until he's home.

The news is different these days. It's been five and half months since we first started hearing about COVID and little over three and half months since the USA declared pandemic. We've all had time to come to terms with the "new normal" as everyone is calling it now. The reports are more commonplace; just part of each day. Less alarming, making it all seem like this is just how it is now. It's grotesque how the numbers don't mean as much anymore—how they're not as shocking. Many have become desensitized to the fact that they aren't just numbers that used to scroll on the bottom of the screen, the numbers are people. And now, it doesn't even make headlines. It's so common that so many people are dying and testing positive each day that it doesn't even warrant top billing on the news any longer. It all feels like they're trying to act as if this is under control and simply a way of life now.

But I have heard the news about the increased "numbers" in the southern states. "Grand Strand [our local hospital] is talking about being at maximum capacity, and worried about staffing and the ability to handle the influx of patients. Of course, Florida is getting redder on the map, showing the rapid increase in cases. It doesn't appear many are taking it seriously. Jordan, our oldest child who calls Florida home, says everything is open and very few are wearing masks.

Scott and I talk about all of that but I change the subject because I'm depressing myself. I tell him that I'm looking forward to us being able to spend time at the beach. The beaches have all opened back up and, since travel restrictions are still in place, the beach is nearly empty. Myrtle Beach, South Carolina, where we live, is a huge tourist destination so the empty beach is a novelty.

"You are going to be so surprised at how blue the water is now. I have never seen it like this. Looks like Caribbean waters. That is the first thing on our list when you get home. Beach day! I can't wait." I tell him, trying to force enough excitement about our plans for the both of us. He's distracted. He's not really listening. This has become more and more common these past weeks. My heart breaks just a little for both of us.

...

The next couple of days go by surprisingly fast. My phone alerts me of a reminder: Last shift. Scott calls on his way in.

"Weird that I'm headed in for the last shift," he tells me. I can hear the complexity of his emotions. He sounds almost sad to be leaving. "I am glad that I will be working it with

Alvin, Kim, Brett, and Shelia, but they are pulling her more to CCU so I may not get to work with her. Will be a good night," he says, trying to be hopeful. "I saw the numbers, 500 more deaths. People think it's slowing, I think it's just resting." He says as if attempting to warn me.

I agree with him. The map is slowly metastasizing red south. I have watched it for months, West Coast, then pops to the northeast, now migrating south, like birds flying south for the winter. I feel it breathing. Getting ready to rage once again. Laughing at all of us for not heeding the warnings, disguising itself, taking advantage of our fear, skepticism, disbelief, and division—using all of it for fuel. Not even close to being done.

"What's for lunch for your last shift" I ask, diverting my own thoughts.

"Steak and eggs, they still laugh at me. But more are asking about it. They think it is funny when we get a pizza and I only eat the toppings and leave the crust. I really believe it's keeping me from getting this shit. I am keeping my inflammation down. Guess I will see. I have antibodies drawn in the morning. Then, I will have my brain tickled for the nasal swab test. So we will know if I have it or have had it."

I always know when he is arriving at work, his voice

changes. His words are the same, but the volume gets low, his words shorter, and the pauses are longer. The space between his "I am here," and his "I'll text when I can," and his "Have a good night," and his "I love you" all get more intense as the days go on. There is a war in those pauses, in the silences between his sentences. He sits in those spaces as a man between. One facing forward into the storm that is still waging inside the hospital walls, and the other looking forward to and missing the calm that is waiting for him at home.

...

The countdown is almost over. T-minus twenty-four hours. My belly butterflies are dancing. I feel uneasy, nervous maybe. A chill comes over me. Scott and I have been together for fourteen years. Have lived a life together, with all the ups and downs, bliss and heartache. I should not be nervous or uneasy to see him. My body knows what my mind hasn't yet accepted. He will be returning home a different man than he was when he left, and I guess that is what makes me nervous. The unknown of who exactly he'll be and who we'll be together and how long it will take for us to intertwine our individual lives again. Regardless, my husband is coming home and that is all that matters right now.

Madison and I spend the entire day and most of the evening crossing off each item on our list to get ready for Scott's return. We tell everyone we see that he's finally coming home. We are giddy with anticipation. When we get home the package he was waiting on is there. I am relieved it arrived and will be here for him when he gets home. Grux and I head to the porch for a final coffee and unwind time. The dim glow of the lights is once again soothing. The coffee tastes good, and gives my soul a warm little hug with each sip. I find myself holding back an audible "ahhhhh".

Grux at my feet, the warmth of his belly feels good on my feet that are aching from shopping all day. The rhythm of his breaths provides a gentle foot massage. I whisper to him, "Daddy is coming home tomorrow. We made it." He stretches deeply, opening his eyes, scooching to reposition. Moments later the silence of the night is filled with his low rumbling snore. I stay on the porch for a while taking it all in. Remembering the last night that Scott was here with me. Remembering the first night I was here without him. And, now, the last night that I'll be here alone. For the first time since Scott left, I feel like I can almost take a deep breath.

The news the next day is wonderful! He got his antibodies

results back. He's never had it. Had his nose violated in the same way that Madison did, except he got a negative result. He is clear to come home. The full-body relief that shudders through me is intense. I gush over text about how excited I am and how happy I am. I almost can't contain myself.

"Honestly, I am shocked that at least the antibodies didn't come back positive with as much as I was in that shit. I mean I wore my stuff like I was supposed to but there were times when you get tired and it hurts and it's so fucking hot, we all would pull our masks down in the break room or bathroom."

He tells me the final few things he has to take care of, plans for getting on the road in the morning, and we get off the phone with fierce, I love yous.. I float through the rest of the day with the hopeful thought of: *Maybe, just maybe, he'll be okay.*

...

Today is the day. I wake early and every cell of my body knows that finally the 131,040 seconds of the thirteen weeks are finally done. All that is left between us is the eleven hour and forty-four minute drive back home. I text him as soon as I grab my phone. He's already on the road.

Deep breath.

Inner squeal.

We did it!

He did it.

We made it.

He didn't get sick.

He survived.

He did it. He did it. He did it.

...

The thing about long drives is that they allow your mind to wander. The radio is on but he's not really listening. In the calm away from the hospital and in the sanctuary of his vehicle, his mind starts replaying scenes from the past thirteen weeks. He was hoping to never recall some of it, having tucked those memories into hidden boxes under lock and key. But they surface regardless as the highway stretches endlessly before him.

He can't help but remember the ages of so many who died. They were his children's ages. Too young. Too healthy. Too much to live for. He remembers every time he had to call the family, how they would beg and plead for him to do everything he could for their son/daughter/sibling. The memories bring the physical sensations back. He feels slick with sweat again, suffocating under the layers of scrubs and plastic and masks. Chills race up his legs as he drives.

He allows the memories to move through him. They won't leave anyway, no matter how hard he tries to force them. They're coming in flashes now. *"I know, you are my friend,"* whispers the El Salvadoran patient who was able to safely come off the vent. Dr. Kochan saying, *"Let's all take a moment and bow our heads."* And now his mind shifts to the gratitude of everyone he worked with. Picturing their faces. Saint Louis, Alvin, Brett, Kim, Shelia, Shaq, LaTasha, Oriana, Donnie. All of them represent grace in his memory reel. He remembers their eyes. How fearful, determined, focused, beaten, and angry they all were. And all their silent tears... Will any of them fully recover from this?

The radio breaks in bringing him back to reality: *As numbers surge, Florida is on target to surpass New York cases for the first time since the start of the pandemic.* His heart picks up its pace, not in anxiety, in preparation. He wipes his face noticing that he too has been silently crying. Not one tear was shed in thirteen weeks, but they are coming in earnest now.

...

Madison and I run around all day getting ready for Scott to arrive. We're even doing our hair and makeup, which for the past few months has not been a priority. A shower was a chore, but today, today is the day. I'm wearing a dress that Scott sent to me for Mother's Day. I've been waiting for a special occasion to wear it and today certainly is that. There is a frenetic energy about the day. Excited. Nervous. Last-minute tasks. He checks in throughout the day sending through a text with each state he enters as he heads south toward home. New Jersey, Pennsylvania, Delaware, Maryland, DC, Virginia, "Fredericksburg, stopping for gas," he sends. With each check in my insides increase activity. He is getting closer. I have replayed this day in my head so many times, the excitement, the tears, the overwhelming relief of him being home and safe and healthy. I've seen through FaceTime how his face has become slimmer. He's lost his tan. But those are the surface-level differences. It's the ones that are deeper that have me nervous.

"SC" my phone alerts us. This is it. He's now in South Carolina. From the border it is only about two hours. Both Madison and I shift into high gear checking everything one final time, wanting it to be perfect for him. Grux and Luna, Madi's french bulldog, are sensing something is happening.

"*Grux, Daddy is almost home.*" His tail nub starts to dance, cautiously. "*Grux, Buddy, it is for real, Daddy's coming home.*" Grux hops around in excitement, moving back and forth from the door to the porch. Luna is running around like she took speed. Our house hasn't felt this much happiness in weeks. Thirteen to be exact.

I check his location. He is five minutes away. Madison and I again run outside to check the decorations we've set-up. The "elmhurststrong" banner is composed of individual flags with the specific letter on each flag, the damn flags keep getting tangled and wrapping the wrong way, so we get tacks, tape, and staples to make sure it stays secure. Taking one last look, I hug her, fighting back my tears.

"He's coming home," I whisper.

Her embrace tightens, "We did it. He's coming home," she whispers back, a reassurance for us both.

Headlights appear. HE IS HOME!

I wait until he parks and opens the door and then fly down the stairs. I leap, trusting he will catch me. He does, of course he does. He always will. He catches me mid flight, the speed and weight keeps the momentum going and we twirl. I have a vice grip around his neck with my arms and my legs wrap tightly around his waist. The emotional dam breaks free. I feel myself unable to hold it back, with every second of the past thirteen weeks releasing itself from my body. I am now ugly crying.

Slowly becoming aware of the world outside the bubble Scott and I are in, I hear Madison laughing. "Mom, you about knocked him down!" shaking her head in happiness at me as she makes her way down to us.

Madi and Scott reunite in such a sweet moment and then we're hurrying things along so we can show him all the surprises we have for him. He isn't moving fast enough so I infuse some urgency into his actions. It feels like he's hesitating, something doesn't feel right. Something is different. I sense it in the energy around us, the way he's moving, the way he's talking. It's those pauses again. I noticed them when we were on the phone, but now they're here too. But, I shove it aside, only wanting to revel in this moment. He is home. That is what matters.

We get inside and Madison and I are talking over each other, word-vomiting thirteen weeks of updates, questions, things we've waited to tell him, neither of us taking many breaths or breaks. He isn't saying much. He isn't reacting either. I hear that damn inner voice again telling me that something is off. We walk him around the outside showing off everything we put together for his homecoming. I feel like a real estate agent at an open house. He doesn't seem appreciative of the decorations, he barely notices. We point them out telling him how funny it was getting the balloons in the car.

"Thank you," he forces out using the same effort to project a smile. I tell myself he's just tired. It's been thirteen weeks of hell plus he's just driven twelve hours. He's just tired, I repeat. I tell him how excited Grux is going to be, and how I have been telling him all day that his Daddy is coming home. He lets a chuckle escape.

When we get inside, Scott heads straight to the bedroom to put his bag down. He doesn't pause, he doesn't acknowledge the bar full of gifts we meticulously put together for him. "GRUX!" he snaps, "let me put my stuff away!"

"Mom, is he sick?" Madison leans over and whispers to me.

When he finally comes out of the bedroom, I look at him. Really look at him. Now that I'm not plastered to his side and my eyes blurry from tears, I see what she's seeing. He is thin, really thin. His neck barely looks strong enough to hold his head. His clothes are baggy. He is pale, sallow. He looks like he just finished a chemo session. His cheeks still have the mask markings, the bridge of his nose pink. His eyes don't smile with his mouth. He can't even force it.

"He's just tired," trying to convince her.

"He's so pale," she continues.

"He hasn't been in the sun for three months so yeah he's lost his tan," still trying to convince us both of something other than reality.

We go through his gifts explaining the thought behind each one. Madison is so excited about the plaque she found. A little wooden desk plaque, painted white with black printing: Not every super hero wears a cape. Some wear SCRUBS. She hands it to him telling him that he is her hero.

He is distant. Awkward. He is distracted. Uncomfortable. "I'm not a hero," he tells her blankly.

Gruxton senses it too. Scott's down on the floor, still awkward, he is unsure of how to play with him. Grux is just as unsure, hesitant, confused. He is so excited to have Scott home, but it is as if they both are meeting for the first time. My inner voice is chiming in again, *He is different.*

I remember his package that was delivered the other day. I get up to hand it to him. He holds it, looking at it for a minute. He then begins unboxing. He removes the plastic bag from the box, gently opens it and sighs. His fingers softly glide across the words COVID on the back. They move in reverence over ELMHURST. As his hands explore the jacket, I see them shake. He ceremoniously puts it on. No words, slowly tears escape, he is remembering. In the same methodical manner, he removes it, placing it on the hanger, positioning it in the closet with honor.

Madison senses the heaviness and retreats to her room. Scott retreats to the porch with his phone. I make us each a coffee and then I join him. Sitting in silence, I can't shake the uneasiness of the night. The last time we were here was the morning he left. We were sad, unsure of what we would both be experiencing over the coming weeks, but we were still us, determined, happy, a unit. This feels very different. Like there is a chasm between us. I want to hear about every single moment. I want to know what he was thinking, feeling, experiencing. I want to bridge the divide between us and be a part of everything that he endured. And I want it all to happen without me having to ask. I don't want to poke or prod. I want him to want to let me in, to bring me into this with him. But we just sit in silence. I am a mix of thoughts and emotions, unable to land on one. I have no idea what he is thinking or feeling. So we continue to sit without saying a word to each other.

"Let's go to bed," he says, breaking the silence.

Heartbroken, confused, frustrated, and honestly disappointed in his indifferent reaction to his homecoming, I agree with him. He pauses at the TV with the remote in hand, as he watches. *"Florida has now surpassed NY in cases."* He says nothing, turning the TV off.

I know this look. He continues to the bathroom, brushes his teeth, kisses me good night. "I love you," he says softly. I snuggle up to him, needing to be physically close to him. I feel his hip bone jab my leg. He is so thin, fragile, almost. We feel awkward, he feels distant. I keep telling myself that he's just tired, he needs time to adjust to being home with us, and that I am making too much out of it. I remember that old saying about things always looking better in the morning. I fall asleep hoping with everything that I am, that it is true.

...

The days that followed Scott's return home were just as unsettled as the day he walked through the door. We tried—I tried, the kids tried, he tried—to resume some version of "normal life" in COVID times. We clung to routines like lifelines: workouts, beach days, dinners together, bedtime rituals. But everything felt fragile. Performative. We were reenacting a life we used to live, hoping it would somehow feel real again.

All of us treaded lightly in his presence. Not out of fear of him—but fear of *triggering* him. We walked on eggshells, careful with our words, cautious with our questions. Not because we didn't want to know, but because we weren't sure we could handle the answers. None of us were prepared to confront the emotions that lingered just beneath the surface. So we prayed we wouldn't have to.

There were moments—fleeting but unmistakable—when I could feel him wanting to release the memories. His body would tense. His eyes would drift. And then he'd start talking.

Conversations with the kids, his mom, even friends would begin casually, but then shift. Suddenly, he was pleading—not for attention, but for understanding. His flashbacks would take over, and his mind's eye would begin to focus on scenes none of us could see. That's when the tears would come. His voice would shake. His leg would start running in place—a nervous tic, a physical manifestation of the trauma trying to escape.

And then he'd stop. Mid-sentence. Mid-memory. No

more words. Only sounds of his tears, and we'd be left in his presence—still, silent, witnessing, trying to imagine what he'd seen. But we couldn't. We *won't* ever be able to. Because no matter how much we love him, no matter how closely we listen, we will never feel the weight of the burden he carries—the burden of being the keeper of so many souls.

He considers three hours of sleep to be "rested", though the darkening halos under his eyes tell a different story. His body is in constant motion–almost frantic. Stillness seems unbearable. The day after he came home, he was already back in the gym. No pause. No rest day. He couldn't wait. He says it's his therapy. And it may be. But what I witness during his workouts tells a different story. Each rep, each set, each drop of sweat feels like a silent scream—a way to push back the memories, the guilt, the grief.

These workouts mirror an internal battle he's trying so hard to deny. He doesn't ease into them. There's no warm-up phase, no graduation of intensity. Instead, it's heavier weights, higher reps, more sets. Another body part. Another, "Just a few more things. I haven't been able to go for three months," he tells me, already an hour and a half in. His voice is casual, but defensive—like he's trying to convince himself as much as me. He leaves the gym saturated, drenched in sweat, his breath ragged, his body exhausted. The release is temporary. The storm inside him hasn't passed—it's just been postponed.

His temper is short now. Unpredictable. The smallest things set him off, and I can't always tell what will do it. Will it be when I forget to take the trash out, or my silly-talk, or Madison sitting on *his* chair on the porch.

Our porch—once a place of calm, of connection—has turned into a space of silent recollection. He sits there, staring into the night, his mind replaying scenes I'll never see. The air feels heavier. The quiet is no longer peaceful—it's turbulent. A reminder that the war didn't end when he left Elmhurst. It followed him home.

When he does talk it is about those he left behind. "I wonder how my Salvadorian patient is doing?" he asks into the dark night. "I hope Shaq and Saint Louis got back safe." Tonight he's scrolling Facebook, "Shaq's baby will be due soon." Talking out loud. "I hope Sheila is doing okay," he continues, continuing his scroll. "These mother fuckers!" an instantaneous shift. "What's wrong?" I ask.

Through clenched jaw he tells me, "Isn't it funny how we have all these funds to make sure police are militarized with all the body amour, riot gear, pepper spray, ammo, weapons, rubber bullets, and whatever they need but nurses didn't have PPE and died because of it." He lashes back. I notice his leg, going a mile a minute, bouncing. He continues. "I take this shit personally," demanding my attention with his glare. "I put myself in this fire to help save lives and there were many we couldn't do anything for. People complaining about wearing a mask, 'Its against my rights,' FUCK you is how I feel. Your rights? It's not over, it's not close to being over, my last shift, four fucking nights ago, I zipped up two more people in body bags." His voice cracks as tears slide down his cheeks.

Trying to comfort him as best as I can, I tell him again, "Baby, I am so so sorry." Honestly, I don't know what to say, or if I should say anything. Do I hug him or just hold his hand? Does he need me to be present but silent? I don't know how to help him.

Unhearing me and continuing to scroll, "Are they not seeing the numbers going up?" His tone sharp. Next comes what I feared most.

"I am going to Florida," he tells me matter of factly.

"What!" I gasp.

"I am going to Florida. Look at the numbers. I talked to some of the nurses I worked with at North Side to check on them, and they are saying it's bad."

I sit and look at him. After the briefest of moments I say: "Well, then I am going too." I tell him just as matter of factly as he told me. "I will contact my recruiter in the morning." Firmly without hesitation I tell him that from now on, where he goes, I go.

I knew he wouldn't argue with me about this. He has become clingy with me. He is with me 24/7. Him not wanting me to do anything without him or vice versa. He may not be talking much, but having me nearby must be healing and soothing for him.

We both land contracts in Florida and find a cute little one bedroom, one bathroom dog-friendly apartment to accommodate Gruxton. We have a week to pack and get there before our start date. Oddly, I am excited. Three months in Clearwater Florida, COVID or not, is going to be beautiful. My excitement though is quickly extinguished.

Scott and I are typically a good team. We rarely argue. Packing is generally a breeze, a coordinated effort making us function like a well-oiled machine. This time was a true test of patience for me. Scott was snappy, opinionated on what I was packing. Irritated, slamming stuff around. Yelling at Gruxton, even. When we pack, Gruxton always knows something is happening. He gets anxious and annoying. Panting, hacking, making sounds like he is about to take his last breath. He is under foot, pacing, trying to dart out the door every time we take something to the car.

And the barking... He starts with a slow short, medium pitch bark-whine combination which quickly turns into loud, high pitch barking. Annoying. Frustrating. Loud. But also something we've come to expect. It happens every time we pack. Only, this time, Scott is yelling at him to stop. Grux just gets louder. It is a chaos fit to send me straight to the loony bin. I'm maxed out. Emotions are too high from being suppressed for too many weeks and in upheaval and confused since Scott came home. I tell them both to shut up. I notice that Grux is acting more anxious than usual though. Realization hits me, he must think Scott is leaving again.

Recognizing this I try to calm him by calming myself and my energy a bit. Scott is completely ignoring it. I tell Scott, "Just stop for a minute, give him love and talk to him, he is feeding off your energy." Scott listens but this just makes Gruxton more excited. This situation is dissolving. Scott is more frustrated and getting angrier. This is not usual. Suddenly all three of us are walking a tight rope. Scott yells as Grux again, enunciating every syllable. Gruxton growls back at him, showing his teeth. I saw the look in Scott's eyes, cold, fury. I immediately grab Grux and wrangle him to his crate and put the blanket over it knowing if I don't diffuse this it will not end well. Scott just grabs up another bin to pack our things in and slams the door as he goes out. What the hell?!?!

It feels like I am living with Jekyll and Hyde. One minute he's flipping off the guy that cut in front of him in traffic. Yelling, "Get off your damn phone and drive," to everyone who has the audacity to be on their phone while driving, i.e., everyone. Then slipping into singing and dancing as if nothing happened and all is good in the world. Yelling angrily at Grux to settle down and then quietly soothing him two seconds later.

Evenings and days off are not a rejuvenating time. Sleep continues to elude him. Gym days are not missed and brutal workouts extend well over two hours. He has radicalized his food regime. I am now a closet eater, sneaking snacks so that I don't disappoint him, or worse, provoke him. He is triggered by everything. I don't think he is even aware. The outbursts are unpredictable, zero to one hundred in seconds without any warning.

...

I remember when he surprised me with my New York City Christmas wish. My heart pounding as the city that never sleeps came into view. Walking through Time Square, the cold air stinging our chest with every breath. We laughed, pointing at every little thing we didn't want the other to miss. We must have said "Look at that!" a million times. The city is living and breathing, vibrant, loud, her crescendo unique. We felt her pulse through our feet, pounding our hearts. I loved her and we made plans filled with wishful promises to return one day. Preferably in the summer next time so our lungs weren't filled with ice. It was magical. Every time I heard something about New York City, or watched a show or movie set in the city, I was transported, reliving Starbucks on Broadway and dancing billboards.

New York City is different now. One of contradiction and confusion. She gave me one of the best memories of my life, only to tarnish it forever. Lady Liberty, now broken, again. I hold a visceral empathy for her. She is weak, her soul heavy, her light, a North Star for so many, dimming slowly, and somehow, she continues to hold up, battered and torn, scarred. She knows better than any of us Scott's haunting cries, "I wish I could've done more," that wake him or prevent him from sleeping. New York has changed, and so has

Scott.

...

"Garrett sent me this," he tells me as he hands me his phone: "Dad, I wrote this song for you after one of our talks while you were in New York." Attached to the text is a video. I push play.

Isolation (Original)- YouTube @garrettmaiers6014

Isolation
Sitting in a room all by yourself
A couple hours might be nice
After a week it feels like hell
And the silence it's deafening.
Only so much one can take
Someone open the door
He's gonna go insane
And I just want you to know that
You did nothing to deserve this
Last week I could see the family and hang with friends
But tonight all alone wondering how's it going to end
And the air it feels so heavy, is this what it's like to drown
It's getting darker, I think the sun is going down

And I just want you to know that you did nothing to deserve this
And nothing scares me more than dying alone.
And nothing scares me more than dying alone.
And nothing scares me more than dying alone.
And nothing scares me more than dying alone.
And nothing scares me more than dying alone.
And nothing scares me more than dying alone.
And nothing scares me more than dying alone.
I just want to see my mom talk to my dad
Talk to any of the friends that I had
So sick of this room. Sick of this pain
Sick of grasping to life, please make this go away
And I just hope that I did nothing to deserve this.

Neither of us have words, only tears. None of them deserved it. Scott didn't deserve this. None of us deserved this.

CHAPTER 14

After the PPE Comes Off

SPRING 2021

What began as running into a calling bigger than him, turned into four more tours after Elmhurst. For over a year he chased COVID, racing to every hot spot—Florida, Texas, and South Carolina. He had one mission: Save people while also relieving burnout or sick nursing colleagues. He continued to chase his mission while running from himself. And for every step into the storm, I was there with him.

Our plans today are beach day. Enjoy being home, back at *our* beach, Myrtle Beach. These are our favorite days. Lazy, warm, endless blue skies, sun belting down on us. UV level of 10 per the certified accurate weather. All of it means one thing: tan lines. Being home in Myrtle Beach is adding icing to the proverbial cake.

Scott took a local contract as a pool ICU float. This is

a new program being implemented by the big hospital in Myrtle Beach. He still is battling COVID amid nursing shortages resulting from COVID.

Zach is now a senior in high school and finally playing baseball again after missing his entire junior year. He sent me his schedule a few weeks ago and he has a game or two that I would be able to make. However, Scott won't because he has to work. How do I tell him I am going? His fuse is so short, and he is more clingy than ever. I know this is going to send him over the edge. As I sit here baking in the sun, running through scenarios in my mind, playing out the conversation, and anticipating his reaction, fully knowing no matter what his reaction is, I must stand firm and go. *Big breath, Jodi.*

"So Zach has a game next week and I want to go since I am able to with my schedule and I haven't been to see him play yet. With COVID already taking so much away from him I feel I need to be there," I try to lean in gently.

"I have to work," he's quick to reply.

"I know I was planning on going up on Thursday and coming back Sunday," quickly dropping my plans on him.

I turn to look at him, nervous, holding my breath and bracing for whatever comes. He loses it. Sobbing, uncontrollably. Noises I've not heard and tremors I've never felt. I get up beside him and pull him to me, wrapping myself around him. He collapses. My worst fears have made their way into the physical world. His spirit and humanness collide back together. No nice meet and greet. These demons he's been fighting against, the ones he has been running from for over a year, have finally caught up with him. They're all escaping his body and he has no control. He sacrificed his body, enduring hospital ICU COVID hell, week after week after week, tour after tour for over a year. Each tour was thirteen weeks. Four completed COVID contracts. Three different strains of COVID, four different states. His eyes forced to see things no one can comprehend, charring and marking his eyes forever. There was no turning away or blinking for him. No hiding behind Facebook posts or pretending it was a hoax. He didn't get the luxury of adjusting to a "new normal" and going on with life. He lived every moment of the pandemic in ways that many will never understand. All of that is violently leaving his body now as we're tangled together on the beach.

The nightly war room collaborations, pleas amongst his fellow colleagues, the video calls he graciously facilitated with families so they could say a final goodbye. He can't unhear those. The feel of his own sweat against his skin for every minute of every hour on his nightly shifts, from the moment he suited up to the final moment he could finally get it all unstuck from his skin. The hands he held, the brows he wiped, the baths he so gently provided, the feel of life leaving, is all branded onto his body. Demanding his own tears not to fall, to stay strong in the face of all the despair. The sting of the mask gripping to his face, the taste of recycled breath dry on his tongue. Each inhale carries the ghost of the day—faint traces of antiseptic, sweat, and sorrow. His ears ring with the whir of machines, the hurried shuffle of nurses, the gasps that cut through the quiet. And always, the scent—not just of disinfectant, but of lives fought for and lost—lodges deep, a haunting reminder that he's breathing in more than air. Despite every effort he tried to escape, suppress, and avoid it all, he couldn't. It crawled on his skin, embedded his thoughts, appeared in his dreams, assumed residence in his heart. Day after day, week after week. He could no longer deny the fragility of his spirit.

There wasn't time for him to feel. He was called again and again to help in any way that he could, and it took such a toll on him. For over a year, there was always someone who needed him to be strong, another alarm to respond to, another incoming patient to care for, another state that was being overwhelmed.

There was the nurse he'd worked beside just the week before—now a patient, eyes wide with fear, asking, "Will I be okay?" And Scott, steady and true, answered, "I will be here either way." It wasn't a promise of outcome. It was a promise of presence.

But that wasn't the only moment that stayed with him. He told me about Christmas Day. A forty-something-year-old mother, intubated, fading. Her family gathered on FaceTime—two small kids, a husband trying to hold it together. Their voices trembled through the screen, offering one last "I love you, Mommy," before the room fell into silence.

And through it all, Scott stood there. In the center of the storm. While the world outside tried to pretend things were normal, he bore witness to the unraveling. To the sacred. To the unbearable.

When he shared these stories, something in me cracked open. I'd heard so many pieces of his shifts—clinical updates, exhaustion, the occasional dark humor—but this was different. This was raw. His voice steady, but something in his eyes gave him away. These moments—her question, his answer, the FaceTime call—had etched itself into him.

I imagined him standing there, mask creased, eyes glassy, holding space for a goodbye no one should have to give through a screen. I remember the weight I felt, trying to absorb what it meant to be the one who stays. To offer presence when certainty is impossible. And I realized, he wasn't just saving lives; he was absorbing grief. Carrying it home in silence. It's moments like these—quiet, unrecorded, deeply human—that shaped the man who returned home to me. Changed. Worn. Still carrying the echoes of those rooms.

These demons slowly took up residence within him, eating at him for over a year. Silently. A little nibble here, a buffet there, gorging themselves until all that remained was the carcass of his spirit—hollowed out, barely recognizable. I watched it happen in slow motion, helpless to stop the unraveling. We were both drowning, just in different ways. And finally, we said it aloud: *We need help.* This was bigger than either of us.

...

Therapy wasn't a fix—it was a lifeline. A turning point. The moment we stopped pretending that grit alone could carry us through. It cracked open the silence we'd been living in, gave language to the pain we'd both been swallowing. For Scott, it was the first time he could lay down the armor, even just for an hour. No ventilators. No war rooms. Just space to feel, to grieve, to begin the long, uneven process of healing.

And for us—our life together—it was a reckoning. Therapy didn't erase the trauma, but it gave us a map through it. It reminded us that love isn't just about surviving side by side; it's about choosing to rebuild, even when the foundation feels scorched. It helped us name the ache. Helped us hold it without being consumed.

It helped *me* help *him*. Because once he found the words, I could finally hear what he'd been carrying. I could meet him in the silence between sentences, in the pauses that used to feel like distance. Therapy gave me the tools to understand his grief without absorbing it, to support him without losing myself. It taught me how to stay present—not just as his wife, but as his witness.

Because the truth is, those moments live in us now. They shaped the way we love, the way we listen, the way we honor what remains. Scott will never be the same. Neither will I. But we're learning to live with the echoes. To find grace in remembering. And even now, years later, we still carry pieces of those patients, those nights, those impossible choices. They're stitched into the fabric of who we are.

And maybe that's the point. Not to forget, but to remember with grace. To honor the staying.

CHAPTER 15

Honorary COVID Angels of Mercy (CAM)

What no one prepares you for, no instructor teaches you, no orientation touches on, no continuing education units [CEUs] acknowledges, is the invisible grief you carry as a nurse. It is tucked away in pockets next to stethoscopes, pens, assignment sheets, cell phones and beepers. It weighs these pockets down, getting heavier every hour of every shift. The expectation? Bear it, quietly, silently, never let it see the light of day.

When our country grew quieter in 2020, there were thousands of nurses who jumped in to help. New York City was recognized as the epicenter, with the highest recorded number of cases and deaths for the year 2020. I am grateful to my husband and his fellow colleagues, especially the Elmhurst COVID warriors, as I have referred to them many times.

This membership is private. They have all earned it through blood, sweat, and so many tears. No one else deserves acceptance into this shared sacred space between them. They know all too well the invisible grief they've been carrying since meeting in 2020. I am grateful to each of them for holding space for my husband. Only they will ever fully understand how this experience has imprinted on him.

They still feel the warmth of their patients' trembling hands, gripped tightly in fear. They still feel those very same hands grow still and loose with no other option but to touch softly. Only they will ever know how it chills your spine when a room full of urgency and chaos suddenly falls quiet and still. Only they know the soul-wrenching impact of that happening every day, on every shift, for weeks and months on end. Only they know the debilitating sound of "I don't want to die" spoken by so many in their final moments. Only they can feel the sting of their heart in finding courage to quiet others' fears, assuring them, *I'll be here either way.* Only they know what it is like to be the custodians of lasts—breaths, touches, goodbyes, prayers. Only they know the ever-lasting burden of being the gatekeepers for all the people who didn't have a choice in any of it.

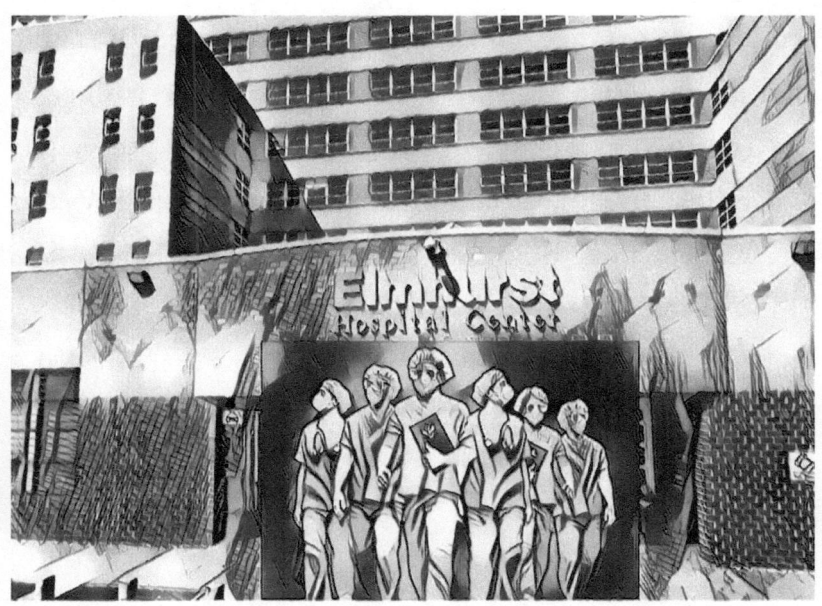

Photo attribution: Background image Google Maps with AI alteration using prompt: Add 6 nurses walking out with masks, 3 female 3 male

The Voices That Carried Us - COVID Angels

What you are about to read are not just stories, they are lived experiences. They are not dramatizations. They are not embellished recollections crafted for effect or coated in insights gained from hindsight.

These are actual words of frontline healthcare workers who served at Elmhurst Hospital at the height of the pandemic. These are the voices of those who stood in the fire when the world was still trying to decide if it was burning.

They did not ask to be heroes. They did not seek the

spotlight. What they did was show up—day after day, night after night—when showing up meant risking everything.

These words are sacred. Unedited. They carry the weight of lives lost, lives saved, and lives forever changed. They are the truth behind the headlines, the humanity behind the PPE, the soul behind the statistics.

Read them slowly. Let them settle. Allow them to shake you. To bear witness is the least we can do. To honor them is the *only* thing to do.

This is their truth.

This is their war.

And this is how they carried us.

Scott Maiers, RN - Travel Nurse, SC

March of 2020: COVID-19 was declared a pandemic. The hospitals where we lived in Myrtle Beach, SC were stopping elective surgeries and census was low. They were laying off nurses. New York City on the other hand was begging for help. That's what I do, I step in and help. I thought with my experience as a Travel ICU RN I could go hit the ground running and really help. I had confidence about my nursing skill set and ability. And I was used to stepping in with little to no orientation as a traveler. I saw on TV the images of NYC and especially Elmhurst Hospital that had been dubbed the

Epicenter of the Epicenter. I called my recruiter and said I need to go to Elmhurst. I didn't hesitate.

I walked into the auditorium on the first day where we got a brief orientation of what to expect and what was expected from us. They told us that day there were over 180 ventilators running. I was stopped in my tracks. On a heavy day most 20 bed units might have 15 or so with patients hooked to it. This was something way outside the norm. We were told where the isolation gear would be and what Level 3 meant. I still felt like "I got this."

During my orientation on the unit, I was with Alvin, a staff nurse at Elmhurst. We would become good friends. The first day I saw patients in their 20's, 30's, 40's and some with no pre-existing conditions. I thought to myself: This isn't the older, more sick people they have been telling us about. I got through the orientation and was back for my first night solo, well nothing was really solo, we had a great team of nurses from all over the country, Alvin (staff at Elmhurst), Sheila (my wife's best friend that I went to New York with), Shaq (from Alabama), Saint Louis (Texas), Kim (Ohio), Brett (Oklahoma), Donnie (Maryland), Oriana (a NP from Colorado), Nicole (Missouri) and Dr. Kochan (Michigan). We became a team, a family fighting against this beast. We helped each other, cried with each other, and held each other up. I will never forget these Angels. My first night, my first patient, went downhill quick. We ended up coding him several times for a few hours. He died. Dr. Kochan stopped everyone and asked us to join hands for a moment of silence for this guy who just died without his loved ones near. I cried then and I still well up at the thought of that moment. That will live with me forever.

It took a toll on all of us. Watching people die without their loved ones, only us by their side, with space suits and gloved hands. It also took a toll on our confidence as medical professionals. Nothing we did was working to save lives, everything we did before, wasn't working. We would stand around each night and discuss what we were going to do, nothing was working. We felt defeated. We didn't have many "wins" but in October, Elmhurst released a video of a patient we had in the unit since March leaving on a stretcher headed to rehab. Every one of us had cared for this man. That felt like a win.

The people of NYC welcomed, encouraged, and cheered for us. Everyone saw the coverage of people hanging out the windows banging pots and pans at 7 p.m. every day. I saw signs in the windows of houses that children had made thanking all the EMS and medical professionals for coming to help. We at Elmhurst also received letters and pictures from elementary school kids from all over the country. I remember one night seeing the ones from South Carolina and I loved that.

The demon at Elmhurst took its toll on us. But we did everything we could to help as many as possible. I took off from NYC to Florida, then South Carolina, then back to Florida, then Texas. After chasing COVID-19, I had to chase my demons. It took its toll on me, I screened for Moderately Severe PTSD. I went through therapy, I did meditation, massages, all the self help things. Therapy saved me. Medical professionals, RN, RRT, physicians, CNA, all the people who worked in this field, especially in Critical Care areas had some degree of PTSD before the pandemic began. COVID made everything worse. I hope that others in this field get the help they so deserve and realize we were not made to see these things and it doesn't make you a weak nurse to get help with it.

Joseph J Kochan, M.D., Captain, Medical Corps, United States Navy

When the author of this book asked me to write a note to myself or to convey some details of my experience in New

York City in the spring and early summer of 2020, I struggled to find words that could express my experience. It has been five years since I first stepped foot in New York City's Elmhurst Hospital, but I vividly remember the 91 days I spent on Active Duty as a Navy Reserve physician. I am and have been an anesthesiologist since 1999, when I completed a Navy residency. In 2001, I left active duty and took a position in the Anesthesiology Department at Sparrow Hospital, a trauma center in Lansing, Michigan, while remaining in the Navy Reserve. It is essential to note that I did not train in critical care medicine. However, anesthesiology is a form of acute critical care medicine, with experience in placing breathing tubes, managing ventilators, and administering intravenous medications that are essential for life support.

It is not, however, intensive care, which is a specialty in its own right, requiring residency training.

On April 2, 2020, I received a call that pulled me and 157 other Navy Reserve physician and nurse colleagues to man Navy Medicine Support Team, Operation Gotham COVID-19 Response, as part of a broader military and civilian operation to assist the overrun New York City Hospital System with the worst pandemic of the 21st Century.

The COVID-19 pandemic hit Michigan in late February

and early March of 2020, with aggressive stay-at-home pro-tocols closing all businesses and schools on March 12th. Sparrow Hospital quickly imposed a moratorium on elective surgeries as the number of hospitalized COVID-19 patients increased. My anesthesiology department continued to man the operating rooms for emergency surgeries and created teams to assist with the massive increase in emergency intu-bations for ventilator support for those in respiratory failure from the COVID-19 virus. On Thursday, April 2nd, while at home awaiting my next shift at the hospital, I received a call from the Deputy Chief of Staff at Naval Medical Forces Atlantic. His order was to review all the medical rosters of the Navy Reserve physicians and nurses from across the United States and determine who was ready to deploy to support a medical response to the COVID-19 pandemic in New York City.

After approximately 36 hours of phone calls, texts, and emails, a list of 157 physicians and nurses was compiled and submitted. By April 4th, we had orders, plane tickets, and transportation arranged to Fort Dix, New Jersey, our entry point into New York City. Our team poured into Fort Dix over the next 48 hours. My journey into this hellish situa-tion started on the morning of April 5th on an almost empty flight from Detroit Metropolitan Airport to Newark. Upon arrival, I was bused to Fort Dix, where I arrived after dark and was housed in an empty barracks room until I was bused with scores of other military personnel into New York City the next morning. I then checked into a hotel in downtown Manhattan, which would become my home for the next three months.

On Monday, April 6th, I met with the other leadership of the Navy Medical Support Team. Two of the other leaders arrived on April 5th and met with Army leadership and the leadership of New York City Hospitals Plus, then traveled to seven of the eleven hospitals in the system. We spent the next 24 hours creating teams of 20-30 nurses and physicians to augment the medical staffs of Bellevue, Elmhurst, Mount Sinai, Coney Island, Harlem, Queens, and Kings County, the areas hardest hit by COVID patients.

Wednesday, April 8th, my team of 28 met at 7:00 a.m. to go to Elmhurst. Once the bus arrived, we were quickly escorted into a large classroom, where we began filling out emergency credential paperwork, received a brief overview of our roles, and were assigned tasks. My assignment would be as a critical care physician manning one of the multiple make-shift intensive care units. Elmhurst had created intensive care units out of multiple regular wards with approximately 180 critical care beds, where almost every patient was intubated and ventilated. I returned that night for a 12-hour shift to train as the sole Navy representative with a traveling critical care physician who was the sole nighttime doctor along with her team of seven, including Elmhurst residents, nurse practitioners, and physician assistants covering approximately 80 patients in the intensive care units including Medical ICU, Cardiac ICU, and a ward that had been converted into an intensive care unit.

The scene was dreadful, with two ventilated patients per room. There were no unventilated patients. We spent the entire night moving from one cardiac arrest to another. By shift change in the morning, six patients had died, three others survived their cardiac arrest, and we admitted six patients from the emergency room. Visiting the emergency room that first night was a frightful scene as we selected the patients to bring to the ICU for care. Not even my deployed time in Afghanistan could have prepared me for the multitude of critically ill patients housed in the ER. There were patients everywhere. Some were sitting in circles around hand-made oxygen splitters that delivered mask and nasal cannula oxygen to up to 10 patients. There were people on gurneys stacked three deep. There was an intensive care unit with intubated and ventilated patients right there in the ER. And due to the overwhelming number of deaths, the morgue was augmented with refrigeration and freezer trucks in the parking lot.

On Thursday, April 9th, I returned to be part of the same ICU Team. The night was quite the same as the first night, with multiple codes, multiple deaths, and multiple admissions. It was then that I learned I would have a team of one intern, two residents, and a nurse practitioner to cover the Medical and Cardiac ICUs, which have approximately 40 beds.

On April 10th and for the next two weeks straight, I worked the 12-hour night shift covering as the critical care physician and lead for my five-person team. As the days passed, the deaths began to decrease, and we cared for a multitude of chronically ventilated COVID patients. After the first two weeks, we stabilized with a slow decrease in new cases, even though Elmhurst remained full, especially in the ICUs. My schedule remained 5 nights out of 7 per week until we started to wrap up our mission at the end of June 2020. There are so many details about this medical mission that I could write about for hours. The COVID pandemic and my time in New York City at Elmhurst will forever be burned in my memory.

My experience was highlighted by the wonderful nurses, nurse practitioners, residents, technicians, and doctors I worked with, including many who were travelers from outside New York, specifically to help care for patients. These included Orianna, Alvin, Shaq, Jodi, Sheila, Brett, Kim, Scott, my Navy colleagues, and so many others. Scott coined the phrase "COVID Angels" to describe the healthcare professionals who graciously cared for those affected by COVID. I learned so much from them, primarily how to counsel families who could not even come to the hospital to see their loved ones, even when they were dying. I cannot thank God enough for those dear friends; I hold them all dear in my heart.

To my fellow COVID Angels, thank you. You will never know how much you kept me in the fight. To my Navy colleagues who risked everything, left their families and homes to go on an unknown and risky mission, I salute you. Most of all, I thank my wife and family for their support. My wife, Alison, spent those 91 days at home alone, unsure of the future, unsure when, or if, I would return. She is my rock and my soulmate.

I dedicate my continued work as a physician to the patients and their families who have been greatly affected by COVID-19.

Alvin Francisco, RN – New York, Staff Elmhurst Hospital

Thanks so much, Scott, for thinking about adding my experience. All I can add is that I am truly grateful to have met some of the best selfless nurses ever and Scott, you, being at the top of the list. You went out of your way and put yourself in harm's way to nurse and help heal patients with COVID-19. The year 2020 was my 18th year of service at Elmhurst hospital center. Throughout those years, I've met a few good nurses. They would come to work, do their thing, complain about short staffing, get paid, and that's it. Then it repeats itself over again. It was like Groundhog Day every day until the pandemic hit and you guys came to help. You changed my whole perspective about fellow nurses, that there are even greater and better nurses out there. You especially were admirable for your bravery in facing the unknown. You actually inspired me to venture out there to other hospitals and help out tackle COVID-19 just like you did. I never thought I could do it, but I did it for 2 years at Jamaica Hospital from 2022 to 2024. I was very much appreciated by the manager and the staff for lending them a helping hand. I felt special and it was an amazing feeling. But I digress, little you know that you actually saved my life.

Remember I was struggling with a fatty liver and hypertension? My doctor was giving me suggestions and prescriptions on what to take but none of them really helped. Had I not met you, my "Keto Guru", I would probably be suffering from cirrhosis by now. Who knows, I probably needed a liver transplant. Knock on wood. With your advice, my LFTs and BP improved because of your advice. I have no one else to thank but you, my friend. To some, you were just a travel nurse sent to Elmhurst Hospital to help with COVID. To me, you were more than that. You were sent here from heaven to help me personally with my own health issues. Because of you, I'm still here fulfilling my mission. You will always be an Elmhurst Strong Hero, Scott. And I'm forever grateful to you my COVID ANGEL friend.

Kim Childress, RN - Travel Nurse, OH

I was working as an ER nurse in Michigan when the pandemic began. It was a horrible flu and RSV season and we had been incredibly busy all winter long. Then February hit and talks of COVID began. We very quickly went from slammed to nothing as people were afraid to come in. The waiting was the hardest part. We heard the stories coming out of New York, we knew it would come for us but not when. I remember my first probable COVID patient, as testing was still not great, who knows if she had it or not. Your mind swirls with wondering if they had it, would I get it, was this the start of it all. We never got "hit" while I was there and as soon as my contract was up, I was on my way to NYC. They were drowning and I could help. I don't know that I had a clue what I signed up for.

It was late April when I got to Elmhurst and I remember my 2 hours of orientation. Doctors and nurses were going from room to room intubating then going back and putting in chest tubes. It felt like a war zone, so completely unlike anything I had ever seen before. Taking care of COVID patients in those early months left me feeling so helpless. As nurses we know what to do when someone can't breathe, how to protect their bodies while intubated, how to protect their brains. None of that worked now. We repositioned their head to try and prevent their ears from breaking down and their oxygen would drop so low and stay there for hours, we didn't dare try and reposition their bodies. Wounds could be healed but depriving the brain of oxygen could lead to irreparable damage. The difficulty in making that choice, of what was an acceptable loss and what wasn't, was not a choice we nurses are used to having to make. Many days it felt like even if we got the patients through all this, their brains would be so damaged from the lack of oxygen they would never have a meaningful recovery. In those early days, I can't remember anyone getting better and leaving. Fighting COVID honestly felt like fighting a war. The fear as it made its way to us, the strength and resilience developed from facing something so hard, and the mental demons left behind. It's five years later and I still cry when thinking about it, although honestly I try not to think about most of it.

I'd be remiss to not talk about the good, as there was some good in all this. I was blessed to meet some of the most incredible people. Working at Elmhurst introduced me to a whole new world of people and I'm better for it. In between changing medications, stabilizing new patients, and banding together to try and save those whose bodies were giving out, we talked and developed friendships that became family. I was blessed to explore New York City without all the people which was both eerie and amazing. I got to explore this normally packed city with an openness and emptiness few will ever experience. There was the 7 o'clock cheer, where people stopped what they were doing to clap, bang pots and pans, cheer and honk; all to thank the medical staff caring for the COVID patients. I still have video of it and I choke up every time I watch it. People stopped me on my way home from work to thank me for being a nurse. I've never seen as much gratitude for the work we did during that time. The best "win" came months later, in October, when Elmhurst shared a video on Facebook. It was of a man leaving the hospital amid staff lining the walls. He was smiling and waving and looked fantastic. This was a man that was in the ICU before I got there, and stayed long after I left. We all took care of him, often doing anything and everything we could to keep him going, many times leaving for the day sure that he wouldn't be there when we returned. Seeing him leave that hospital, the big smile spread across his face, was the moment it all felt worth it. As nurses we all have patients that we will never forget, that stay tucked in our hearts for our entire career. This man will forever be in my heart, he will always be with me to remind me that even when it's hard and seems hopeless, there is reason to keep going. What we do as nurses and doctors matter.

Oriana Cruz, NP - Travel Nurse Practitioner, CO

Note to self,

 This traumatic, harrowing experience will forever alter

your path in healthcare. You took care of community members, most likely recent immigrants, in Queens, NY that had inadequate access to healthcare as evidenced by undiagnosed or untreated comorbidities. Remember all those phone calls you made in Spanish? But guess what? It does get better! You transition to caring for indigenous people.

Per the IHS website, "The American Indian and Alaska Native people have long experienced lower health status when compared with other Americans. Lower life expectancy and the disproportionate disease burden exist perhaps because of inadequate education, disproportionate poverty, discrimination in the delivery of health services, and cultural differences. These are broad quality of life issues rooted in economic adversity and poor social conditions."

The COVID crisis health care providers and my patients will forever be enmeshed in my life, kinda like scar tissue. Formation of scar tissue is a part of the body's healing process. I still have a lot of healing to do, but it's a start.

Shelia Arruda, RN - Travel Nurse, SC

An Oath. A calling. A promise. A pledge. It's who we are. It's what we do. Dedicate our lives to saving you. Once upon a time, in a city that never sleeps, was a family I never knew I had. You see, the end of March 2020 when I lost my wings to return to my roots is where my story began. I called my mom like I always do. I said, "Hey I'm thinking of coming home for Dad's birthday." I was living in Myrtle Beach at the time. Home is Rome, NY. Mom said, "Haven't you seen the news? COVID cases are on the rise. Cuomo is bringing in the Navy ship, there aren't enough supplies. The world is in crisis, there's a full blown pandemic." I laughed and said, "Ma C'mon. How bad can it be? The flu is a virus, the GI bug, HIV, TB. This will be no different than that."

From the moment, sitting in my bubble bath, phone in hand...I googled Manhattan, Brooklyn, the Bronx, NYC. I knew then and there it's where I had to be. I called my husband, my ex, my best friend... and I told them, ready or not, I'm taking a COVID contract. I don't know what it means or what it entails, but with one foot in ICU and another in Hospice, how bad can it be? My best friend says to me, "Don't tell Scott." But, Scott, as he is, with ICU/Hospice ESP, calls and says he's going to Elmhurst with me. Just my COVID Cloud Warrior Buddy and me. He packs up our stuff and drives the Jeep. I go to Charleston, hug my babies, cry, and say one last good bye. I board a healthcare heroes flight to JFK. The plane was silent. It was still. We arrived, planes lining the empty tarmac. No people, no crowds, no music, no smells, no sights, no city lights. Just "thank you heroes," clanging pots and pans at 7 p.m. every night, and refrigerated tractor trailers... containing someone's someone. Scott and I walked to and from work every night, most times not saying a word, sometimes just talking out the night we had, scheming, and plotting, brainstorming, all the whys and what ifs. What happens if we get sick? What happens if we don't make it back? Take the anxiety, the fear, the excitement, and the pure adrenaline and intensify it.

There are still events that even now, five and a half years later, I can't disclose. I don't want to talk about...because every night, every hour, it was code after code. COVID didn't discriminate—young or old, male or female, petite or full figured, we were there. We showed up time and time again, to give those before us some reprieve, a moment to breathe, a chance to take a minute for basic human needs.

We fought the unknown side by side. States across the nation, healthcare professionals from every specialty determined to fight the battle and save at least one. It didn't matter to us if you came from a penthouse in the sky or a shack by the sea, what your political views were, socioeconomic status was, or how you identified. Our job was to treat you just the same, save your ass, or just be a gloved hand to hold yours at the end. Airway protected, mechanically ventilated, blood pressure supported, in room HD, full code or DNR/DNI, we were your voice.

So what happens when everything we were trained to do just doesn't work this time. What do we do when you're the same age as us, as our friends, as our families, and we have to say goodbye. There isn't a provider in this book that will say we didn't try. Sometimes we would just look at each other and cry—no explanation needed, like a weight was lifted and only we knew why. We didn't talk to our families, it was our way of protecting and preserving their innocence. Most times, we couldn't laugh, we couldn't cry... we were drained, exhausted, defeated, and lost a sense of pride when our skills just didn't work.

Oh, but we embraced every glimmer of hope we were given. Did you see that *he wiggled his toes, she squeezed my hand, he's breathing over the vent and fighting it?* Every milestone is a miracle—we were like proud parents protecting our babies. I don't know if y'all have ever met an ICU nurse, but we are pretty territorial! We took turns watching each other's patients, even the nights we were off we couldn't flip the switch, couldn't separate, and would text each other with updates. We'd talk to you, sing to you, pray with and for you. We'd put you in a hammock (the hoyer lift) and bring you to the window, tubes, lines, and all...just to get you out of that bed because 2 months before we were assembling a team to turn you like a well-oiled machine, code after code. Our movements in sync, our eyes said all that our voices couldn't. Most of you won't remember our names but we will never forget your face and within us, there will always be this place.

To my friends that become family: we have one hell of a story, one unbreakable bond, and I thank you. Without you, I wouldn't be the me that I am today. Where the whistle of a train brings me more peace than I've ever known because in the darkness of every night, there's a reminder that there's still a light.

- Shelayla aka Backpack

Brett Locke, NP, RN - Travel Nurse, OK

Volunteering at Elmhurst Hospital in New York City during the height of the COVID-19 pandemic was one of the most profound experiences of my life. Working in the ICU alongside critically ill patients, I witnessed both unimaginable loss and extraordinary resilience. Despite the overwhelming circumstances, the staff welcomed us with open arms. The nurses and team at Elmhurst showed a level of strength, compassion, and unity that I will never forget.

What began as a call to serve quickly turned into something much deeper. I formed bonds with colleagues that will last a lifetime. In the darkest of days, we found light in one another. I am incredibly grateful for every person I worked with during that time. Elmhurst was truly ground zero, and yet in the middle of so much pain, there was also so much humanity. It was a privilege to stand beside such courageous people.

Nicole Duckwall, RN - Travel Nurse, MO

COVID-19 was no joke and it was real! Upon arrival we were greeted then shuffled into a large room for a quick safety brief and given our assignments. Then we spent a couple hours shadowing a nurse on the unit where we were assigned. It was very apparent the staff were overwhelmed and exhausted. Those of us assigned the night shift were sent back to our hotels with instructions to return at 6:45 p.m. for our first of many nights. The day-shifters stayed and were immediately assigned a preceptor for the first 2 hours of their shift. During our safety briefing we were told one of Elmhurst's own nurses and a supply tech had recently died as a result of COVID and many of the staff had lost multiple family members as well. The staff appeared shell-shocked and were very apprehensive to go into their patients' rooms for fear of contracting COVID and or passing it on to their loved ones and friends. Most nurses were staying in hotels and not going home in between work shifts.

The ER was overflowing but the patients could not be admitted to the units until there was a bed made available. During the height of the pandemic, patients were not surviving. It was not uncommon to hear "code blue," insert any unit, called multiple times each day and night, with none surviving. Patients on gurneys were lined up in the hallways waiting for the previous patient to be declared deceased, tagged, and removed from the room. Once the room was deep cleaned and sanitized with the special UVC (ultraviolet C) lights, they would become the next occupant.

My first night on the unit we had 3 codes, none of which survived. This was a real gut punch and a reality check that we were in it for the long haul. I quickly came to realize why New York was begging for travel nurses from all over the United States. They were drowning with no end in sight. Bodies were stacking up in the refrigerator trucks behind the hospital. Elmhurst is a hospital in Queens, one of the poorest, hardest hit boroughs of New York City, yet they never turned anyone away because they are a city hospital. People had been told to shelter in place but this only exacerbated the situation as many homes were multi-generational, thus the virus killed off entire families. Many waited until it was too late to seek medical attention as they were already coughing up black-tar sputum, their lung x-rays described ground glass opacities and oxygen saturations were below 60%, unsustainable for life.

Night after night the same scene played all throughout the hospital. Before COVID, Elmhurst was a level one trauma center with many specialties to include pediatric and neonatal. All patients other than adults were transferred out and Elmhurst became one of many COVID designated hospitals in New York City. All ventilators were in use, including transport vents. The hospital was in such high need that ventilators had to be shipped in. Medications were in short supply and we were forced to mix our own drips and calculate the concentrations and enter them into the IV pumps. Propofol was out on the counters and narcotics were in the locked box in the medication room. We had to find the medication nurse for the shift (hospital staff) so she could use the key and unlock the meds, which we signed out on using pen and paper. Elmhurst did not have a Pyxis system to manage and keep track of medications to include narcotics.

We learned to rely on each other, especially at night

because we had less staff. I made some lifetime friends while working at Elmhurst. I was living in a hotel in Manhattan and commuting by subway to Queens every night I worked. I had never ridden on the subway prior to this travel assignment and it took some getting used to. Everything was shut down, all restaurants, all federal and state buildings, all churches, and pretty much everything except necessary services. Famous chefs prepared nutritious meals and donated them for the health care workers since their restaurants were closed. These meals were handed out upon our arrival and we received breakfast when we left in the morning for the entire first month we were there.

Elmhurst had a prone team (U.S. Military) that would come like clock-work to either flip our patients prone, where they would remain for 16hrs, or supine for 8 hours, for a total of 24 hours. This team worked in sync like a well-oiled machine. They were very methodical, meticulous, and moved quickly from room to room. Patients' family members were not allowed in the hospital, so when it came time to say their final goodbyes, I would take my phone into my patient's room and call their family and place my phone (in its protective pouch) upon their pillow so they could hear their loved one's voices. There were many times these calls lasted greater than 30 minutes. Sometimes, family would read scripture, sing, talk, or play a favorite song.

I wore my N95 mask for nearly three weeks before the hospital started receiving new masks and additional PPE (Personal Protective Equipment). After this we were able to change our N95 masks out every 2 to 3 days unless it was visibly soiled. We would arrive to work about 15 to 20 minutes prior to shift start, sign in, go to the breakroom to drop off our food and bags and don the PPE outside of the unit. We would put on the plastic white hazmat suits over our uniforms, a paper liquid repellent gown, a hair net, shoe covers, goggles, and a face shield. Then we would don our N95 mask with a regular patient mask placed over it and finally we would double glove for extra protection.

May 9, 2020 was a somber shift. This was the night that one of Elmhurst's own beloved Paramedic/Firefighter was removed from life support after losing his battle with COVID. I was working on the 7th floor and just after 8 p.m., ambulances and fire trucks were paired two deep and lined the streets in front of the hospital and for several blocks surrounding the hospital. The lines of emergency vehicles with lights and sirens blaring seemed to never end. That moment seared into my brain as everything became very surreal.

This hero in top shape and only a few years younger than I, had succumbed to the Corona Virus. He left behind a wife and 4 children. It was this moment that I realized I was not immune to its grasp and I so badly wanted to return home to my husband, children, and extended family safe and healthy. I took a picture with Tameka, as we sat in the window sill on the 7th floor looking down at all the emergency lights. We must have cried for 20 minutes.

While at Elmhurst riots broke out, mostly spearheaded by Black Lives Matter (BLM) and Antifa. The morning of June 1st 2020, I observed graffiti all along the streets, broken glass and destruction in the subway stations and a multitude of torched cars, some still on fire lined up and down the street of the hotel I was living in and the Empire State Building. I walked into the hotel to find the front desk clerk frantic and in tears and boards being placed over the windows. She stated, "They tried to kill me and burn down the hotel." Her boyfriend picked her up and when they started to drive, the crowd of protesters started rocking their car and would not let them pass. She remained visibly shaken until she called her boss and he allowed her to go home. Fortunately, my friend Melissa and I had already signed a lease to move out of the hotel and into an apartment across town that very morning. The apartment had an accessible rooftop that allowed us to see the entire downtown of Manhattan.

To be honest, there were times I was more afraid of the riots than COVID. I didn't dare tell my husband or he would have insisted I end my contract and come home early. In addition to the riots, Elmhurst was threatened with bomb threats and some hospital staff were sent death threats. For a short time we were advised to NOT wear our nursing uniforms for our safety. Nurses were getting jumped and assaulted on their way to and from work, both on the streets as well as on the subway.

I made many friends that I still keep in touch with 5 years later, some I know will be friends for life. We had some crazy times and experienced some very physically and emotionally difficult times, some of the more traumatizing memories haunt me to this day. However, looking back, I would not trade any of these experiences, good or bad, because they helped shape me into the nurse I am today. I will never forget: Melissa, Alvin, Scott, Mia, Oriana, Kim, Sheila, Tomeka, Dr. J. Kochan (USN), Respiratory Therapists and so many more that accepted me and treated me like family and took me under their wing and mentored me in all things COVID-19. I also appreciate the chance to teach and mentor other less experienced nurses, all things Critical Care. We all share a bond because we served together and that is what makes us ELMHURST STRONG!!!

Latasha Young, RN - Travel Nurse, TX

March 30, 2020 I flew to NYC to help those in need, to be a servant, to further live in my purpose. I came to help and I came to make money. I didn't come to make memories or friends. I came to work, packing every navy blue scrub I owned and harassing TCs for more.

However, I have created memories, I have made life long friends and I WERKED...I love dialysis but baaabbyyyyy ya girl got muscles from pushing those machines. When the doctors and staff saw us coming with those machines, they sighed in relief knowing and believing this treatment was going to help the patient, and for most of them it did.

I've never been in a war, but when I first came to Elmhurst, it was nothing I could have pictured. It was like a war zone. There were bodies, many of them. It was fear, it was sadness, it was a lot of the unknown. It was ALL hands on deck! I witnessed so many people leaving this world to enter their resting place. I witnessed patients transition from ICU to medical floors, getting well and progressing. I also witnessed social workers doing FaceTime calls to families to give updates and letting them see their loved ones. I saw patients get better, I saw the staff getting well and returning to work, I saw ALL people working in unity. Doctors actually listening. I didn't see anything that resembled racism!!!!!!

"We are here putting our lives on the line," someone said. I didn't think of it that way. I was coming to help, but in a sense we put ourselves in harm's way to do our duty. To keep others safe. We've had to celebrate our families birthdays, anniversaries, GRADUATIONS from afar. Families, I hope y'all truly understand that we were there in spirit and thank God and Apple for FaceTime.

I pray my son truly understands why I wasn't there to see him receive his diploma. Cario, I'm exceedingly proud of you and I pray you become the most awesome man I've ever known and raised. Yes, the bar is set high, Son.

After 98 nights I can say this, NYC was doing better.

I remember us all getting on the bus and trying to get in any and all talk time with our loved ones while on our 30-45 min ride. I remember holding patients' hands so they didn't die alone. I remember having bad days, being tired, fatigued, sleep deprived, hungry; but I also remember us laughing, praying for this disease to go away, helping make a difference, enjoying each other, having fun when we could. I remember what it was and how it is now. I saw every RN, PA, NP, LPN, housekeeper, cafe workers, RT, MD, PCTs, and military put their 10000000000000% into helping make a difference at Elmhurst Hospital and we did.

Elmhurst I love you guys and I pray things only continue to get better for you all and the patients. Thanks for receiving me. Thanks for being so appreciative of our help!!!!! I'm forever grateful to have received so much love from you guys.

Thanks to my family and friends: You guys supported me, checked on my kids, sent donations, listened to me vent, prayers. I appreciate everything you guys did.

WITH GRATITUDE

Scott Maiers, RN, ICU—my husband, my hero. Your bravery in COVID's darkest hours became the fire that kept this story alive, even when I doubted my voice. You didn't just fight a virus–you fought for humanity, dignity, and for every breath that could be saved. Your courage to admit when you weren't okay has shaped every page. You have always been *enough*. I love you.

Our six children—who sacrificed their dad so that others might live. When the world applauded and spewed on the frontline, you lived the cost of it. You watched us both unravel and still stood by us with love, steadying us with your quiet strength and unwavering grace. You carried more than your share–holding space for our grief, while masking your own. You didn't ask for this, but you rose to meet it. Your resilience and love is woven to every page. This story belongs to you, too.

Gruxton, our beloved English bulldog—For 11 years and 4 months, you were more than a pet. You were part of our heart beats, our laughter, our healing. You gave us slubber kisses when we needed comfort, tail nub wriggles when joy overflowed, and stink-eye looks that spoke louder than words. You knew us. You loved us. And we loved you right back. You were there through the chaos, the quiet, the porch talks, and the tears. You were family. You still are. We miss you every day. And we feel you still—in the soft thud of memory, the way love lingers long after goodbye.

Sheila—true friend and fellow nurse—who held Scott's hand when I couldn't, and who listened to every fear I dared to share.

My Dad and Sally-Dad, you don't just root fro me-you raised me, in every sense of the word. You showed up as both mother and father, filling the gaps with love, wisdom and steadiness that shaped the woman I am today. Thank you for your steadfast faith in me. You are the kind of dad whose strength lives in the background, but whose love is woven into the way I show up in the world.

Jackie, my sister-thank you for showing up for me. When I couldn't look on the bright side, you sat with me in the dark. Just like the quote from *Alice in Wonderland*-you didn't force light, you were the light by staying. I love you.

Momma Jo, Scott's mom-your love has always been fierce, protective and deeply felt. During the darkest days you carried a mother's fear with grace. You learned to be proud through the worry, to trust Scott's calling even when it terrified you. You never asked for recognition, but you deserve it. Because behind every brave nurse is a mother who taught him how to care, how to endure and love without condition.

To the Elmhurst COVID Angels–Thank you for showing up when the world cried. Through Scott's stories of those darkest hours I saw your courage, heartbreak and compassion. You are etched into our story, our hearts, carrying a legacy of what it means to truly care.

To Michael Allen, author and a relentless encourager— You listened to my story pitch when it was still just a fragile dream. For five years, you reminded me—again and again— to *get this story out*. You believed in its power before it had pages, and in me before I had the courage to write them. Thank you for seeing this story when it was still invisible. For holding space for its becoming. For encouraging me to bring it home.

To Michelle Ireland, editor and publisher—You are not what I expected in this space—and that's what makes you extraordinary. You didn't just edit my words; you heard my heart. You saw the vision tucked behind the grief and pushed me to write with more honesty, more depth, more courage than I thought I had.

Your guidance challenged me to go to places I'd long avoided, to unearth emotions I'd long tucked away. You asked the hard questions, held space for the messy answers, and never let me settle for surface when depth was calling. Thank you for honoring the truth. For helping me bring this story into the world with integrity, courage, and grace.

To all frontline nurses and healthcare workers still carrying the echoes: You are seen. You are remembered. You are never alone. It's okay not to be okay. I salute you.

To you the reader–Whether you've lived this story, loved someone through it, or are just beginning to understand its weight—thank you for bearing witness. May these pages remind you that healing is not linear, that presence is powerful, and that the quiet acts of staying are what shape us most.

CARING FOR THOSE WHO CARE FOR US

The mental health of those in charge of our most human needs and care must not be neglected. Anything less than system-wide embrace of this ideology intentionally neglects every patient and every caregiver.

In an effort to demonstrate due care with more than words, Arching Foundation, a 501(c)(3) nonprofit, will proudly fiscally sponsor selected applicants who demonstrate that they are up to the task of positively contributing toward greater mental health support for the nursing community.

- Brian J. Davis, CEO of Arching Foundation, Inc., a 501(c)(3) nonprofit www.ArchingFoundation.org

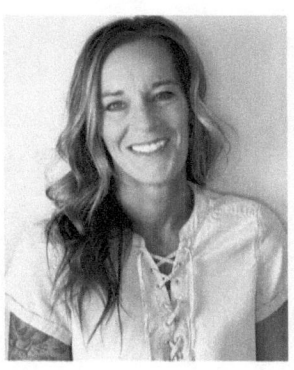

ABOUT THE AUTHOR

Jodi Maiers is a registered nurse with over 15 years of experience, including 12 years in hospice and her current work as a travel nurse. Based in Myrtle Beach, South Carolina, she brings both professional insight and personal depth to her writing. As the wife of an ICU nurse who served during the height of COVID, Jodi witnessed firsthand the emotional toll of frontline care—and the silent impact it leaves on families. Her debut book, *13 Weeks*, is a powerful memoir that invites readers to reckon with the unseen cost of caregiving, both inside and outside hospital walls. A mother of six grown children, Jodi is passionate about creating space for healing through honest conversation, emotional permission, and shared truth. You can connect with her and learn more about her work at Jodi Maiers on FaceBook. j_maiers on Instagram. Email: jodimaiers_author@outlook.com

Soul Spark
— PUBLISHING —

Ready to share your story with the world?

If something in this book made you pause—that quiet moment of *"I could tell my story too"* or you heard the whisper of *"maybe it's my turn,"* take this as your sign to begin.

At Soul Spark Publishing, we believe stories shape the way we understand ourselves and each other. Yours is no exception— and it deserves to be guided with expertise, intention, and a whole lot of heart.

Whether you're drawn to write a memoir, capture a legacy, or shape your lived experience into story-first nonfiction, we'll walk beside you every step of the way.

Our collaborative publishing journey is intentionally small, deeply personal, and grounded in one simple truth: books can change lives—starting with the author's.
If that feels like your next chapter, we'd love to help you begin.

soulsparkpublishing.com
Your story is worthy. Let's bring it to life..

www.ingramcontent.com/pod-product-compliance
Lightning Source LLC
Chambersburg PA
CBHW021221130626
46554CB00004B/1318